THE
TOP 100 RECIPES
for a healthy
LUNCHBOX

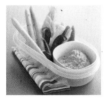

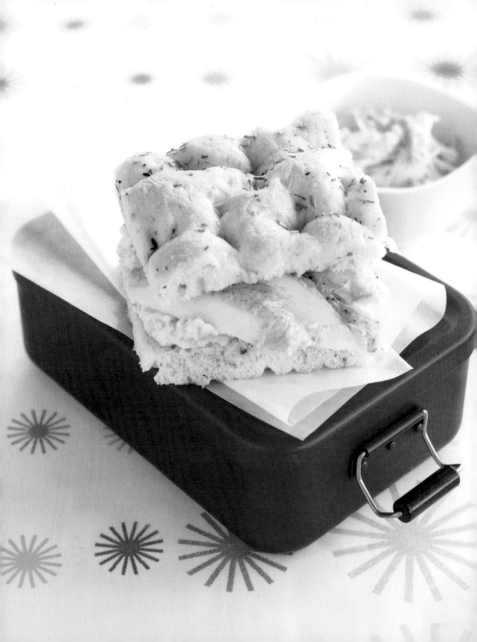

THE
TOP 100 RECIPES
for a healthy

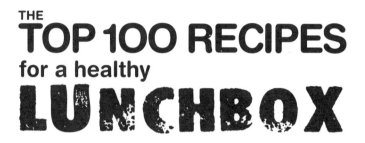

Nicola Graimes

EASY AND EXCITING IDEAS FOR YOUR CHILD'S LUNCHES

DUNCAN BAIRD PUBLISHERS
LONDON

The Top 100 Recipes for a Healthy Lunchbox
Nicola Graimes

First published in the United Kingdom and Ireland in 2007 by
Duncan Baird Publishers Ltd
Sixth Floor
Castle House
75–76 Wells Street
London W1T 3QH

Conceived, created and designed by
Duncan Baird Publishers

Managing Editor: Grace Cheetham
Editor: Alison Bolus
Managing Designer: Daniel Sturges
Commissioned photography: David Munn
Food stylist: Bridget Sargeson
Prop stylist: Wei Tang

British Library Cataloguing-in-Publication Data:
A CIP record for this book is available from the British Library

ISBN: 978-1-84483-517-1

10 9 8 7 6 5 4 3 2 1

To Ella and Joel
**I would like to thank Grace Cheetham for
commissioning me to write this book. My
appreciation also goes to Alison Bolus for her
meticulous editing, and the team at DBP.**

Typeset in Helvetica Condensed
Colour reproduction by Colourscan, Singapore
Printed in China by Imago

Publisher's Note
The information in this book is not intended as a substitute for
professional medical advice and treatment. If you are pregnant
or breastfeeding or have any special dietary requirements or
medical conditions, it is recommended that you consult a
medical professional before following any of the information
or recipes contained in this book. Duncan Baird Publishers,
or any other persons who have been involved in working on
this publication, cannot accept responsibility for any errors
or omissions, inadvertent or not, that may be found in the
recipes or text, or for any problems that may arise as a result
of preparing one of these recipes or following the advice
contained in this work.

Notes on the Recipes
Unless otherwise stated:
Use medium eggs, fruit and vegetables
Use fresh herbs
Do not mix metric and imperial measurements
1 tsp = 5ml   1 tbsp = 15ml   1 cup = 250ml

Symbols are used to identify even small amounts of an
ingredient, such as the seeds symbol for sunflower oil. Dairy
foods in this book may include cows', goats' or sheep's milk.
The vegetarian symbol is given to cheeses made using
vegetarian rennet. Please check the manufacturer's labelling
before purchase, since some brands may vary. Ensure that
foods are kept chilled until the time of eating, where possible,
and that only the relevantly identified foods are given to those
children with a food allergy or intolerance.

contents

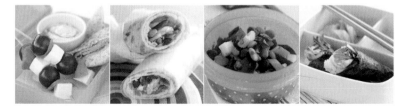

KEY TO SYMBOLS

Ⓥ Suitable for vegetarians: These recipes contain no animal produce, and so can be a good choice for children suffering from inflammatory conditions, such as eczema, asthma and acne, and digestive problems.

Ⓖ Gluten-free: Gluten is the substance in wheat, rye, barley and oats that adds "stickiness" to baked goods. Gluten intolerance may cause inflammation, depression and digestive problems. Gluten-free grains include buckwheat and corn.

Ⓦ Wheat-free: Wheat can be difficult to digest. Replace it with corn, buckwheat, rice, tapioca and rye flours. You can buy wheat-free breads, wraps and pizza bases.

Ⓓ Dairy-free: Milk can be the cause of nasal blockages and sinusitis, catarrh, and throat and chest infections. It may also trigger conditions such as asthma, eczema or acne. Try rice, almond, oat or soya milk.

Ⓔ Contains eggs: If your child has an egg intolerance, it is especially important to give them fresh foods, as egg is often used commercially as a binding agent and thickener. Substitutes for baking are made from arrowroot and agar agar.

Ⓝ Contains nuts: If your child has a nut allergy, you can substitute nuts with seeds that you know your child can eat. Never give whole nuts to children under 5, as they can cause choking.

Ⓢ Contains seeds: Pumpkin, sesame, sunflower and hemp seeds are highly nutritious, but some seeds, particularly sesame, can cause an allergic reaction and so your child may need to avoid them.

INTRODUCTION

For one reason or another, packed lunches seem to throw many of us into a state of panic. The combination of lack of time, early mornings and a desire to produce a lunch that is varied, interesting and nutritious and that's not going to come back untouched can be just too much to contemplate five days a week. It's all too easy to slip into a rut when filling a lunchbox, but with a little forward planning and the help of the 100 recipes in this book, you should be inspired.

Lunch is an important meal for everyone but particularly for children, who have high energy requirements for their size. This means that they need nutrient-dense foods in small, regular amounts to keep their bodies and minds working at their

best. New evidence suggests a correlation between a child's diet and academic performance. Poor diet is likely to lead to a child with concentration problems, memory difficulties, irritability and an increased susceptibility to colds and illnesses. By contrast, children who eat regular healthy meals tend to have more energy, improved learning and a lower obesity rate.

Tempting as they are, try not to rely on the plethora of pre-packed, processed foods specifically aimed at children's lunchboxes. Most of them are wasteful owing to excessive packaging and also contain high amounts of salt, saturated or hydrogenated fat, sugar, additives and preservatives; it will come as no surprise that these foods have a negative effect not only on our children's health but on the environment too. It's all too easy to get sucked in by their overwhelmingly colourful presence in supermarkets. Recent research in the UK found that only one in five lunchboxes is healthy enough to meet Government standards, and the UK is not alone in this situation.

ABOUT THIS BOOK

The main aim of this book is to inspire. The majority of the recipes are quick and easy to prepare; others take a little more forethought and preparation but can be made in bulk and frozen for future use. Many of the recipes will also keep for a few days in the fridge, allowing you to plan ahead and ease the morning pressure.

The emphasis is on good-quality, wholesome fresh food without being puritanical – you will find, therefore, some recipes for sweet treats. Many of these contain fruit; try to avoid giving those that

don't to your child every day, although it's not necessary to avoid them altogether – there's nothing more tempting than a food that's not allowed! The same goes for crisps – give them as an occasional treat and choose brands that are made with good, honest ingredients, avoid overly coloured snacks and steer clear of those that contain a long list of additives. You will notice that the recipes in this book are not full of suggestions to switch to low-fat this or "lite" that. Why? Because many of these foods may indeed be lower in fat than the original article, but they invariably contain additives to compensate for the lack of taste. A food is not necessarily healthy just because it's low in fat and, strangely, some low-fat foods contain bucketloads of sugar. Obviously our children's diets should not be overloaded with saturated or hydrogenated fat, sugar and salt, but it's equally important to eat foods that have been produced with care and consideration, such as free-range, organic and Fairtrade foods.

Each recipe comes with an explanation of its health benefits as well as some serving suggestions, enabling you to create a nutritionally balanced and varied lunchbox on a daily basis. Use the serving suggestions as a guide: you don't have to stick to them religiously, as obviously likes and dislikes as well as the foods you have to hand will influence what you decide to pack in the lunchbox. As for portion sizes, these are averages only, as the size of meals you need to make will obviously differ widely depending on whether you have a picky five-year-old or a ravenous teenager.

The recipes have been created to appeal to both adults and children. While being devised as part of a packed lunch for a child, they could equally be taken to the office, form part of a picnic or be eaten at home for lunch; many of the recipes would also make a welcome after-school supper.

SPECIAL DIETS

If your child is a vegetarian or vegan, has an allergy to nuts or an intolerance of dairy products, eggs, wheat or gluten, you will need to take more care when preparing their lunchboxes. The symbols shown on page 6 are used throughout the book to indicate which recipes are safe for particular diets, and the menu plans provided on pages 140–143 give ideas for a week's worth of lunchboxes for some of these diets.

PLANNING AHEAD

A little forethought makes preparing a lunchbox so much easier. Not only does it relieve the daily panic of what to include, but it also makes the weekly shop more straightforward. This is the perfect time to get your child involved too by giving them the opportunity to choose foods that they would like in their lunchbox, on the premise that they are more likely to eat what they have selected or helped to prepare.

Write down a daily menu for the week ahead, referring to pages 140–143 for guidelines or to use as a template. The menu can be made up of fresh fruit and vegetables, freshly prepared foods, and some pre-prepared and frozen dishes, as well as those invaluable leftovers.

When you are deciding on what to cook for dinner, think how you can incorporate leftovers into a lunch the following day, or just cook a bit extra. The following foods have potential as leftovers and make excellent additions to a lunchbox:

- Pasta, rice, potatoes, couscous, bulghur wheat or pearl barley (although note that you should keep cooked rice and grains for no longer than two days in the fridge to avoid any danger of food poisoning)
- Meat and poultry – chicken, turkey, beef, lamb or pork, or any type of sausage
- Fish and shellfish – grilled/griddled tuna, salmon or trout, prawns or squid
- Vegetables – roasted or grilled

- Eggs – soft or hard boiled, omelette, frittata or tortilla
- Undressed salads
- Soup
- Fruit – sauces, compotes, salads.

CHOOSING A LUNCHBOX

There is plenty of choice when looking for a lunchbox, and your child will probably want to be involved in choosing their favourite, whether it be an attractive colour or decorated with a popular cartoon character. It's an important consideration to make, as a lunchbox can often make or break the success of a packed lunch – an embarrassing, age-inappropriate design is simply not "cool" enough to be seen with!

- Make sure the lunchbox is sturdy, the handle is strong enough to withstand being swung around, and the box can be opened and closed easily by a child.
- Ensure the lunchbox is insulated and/or comes with an ice-pack if your child does

not have access to a fridge at school. This is important for cooked meat, eggs, dairy foods, seafood and rice, couscous and bulghur wheat salads, which should all ideally be kept cold until lunchtime. Many lunchboxes come with a separate pocket or section in which the ice-pack can be inserted so that it doesn't come into contact with the contents.

- Make sure the lunchbox is large enough to hold a drink bottle, or a flask for winter months. Warm the flask first by filling it with just-boiled water for 15 minutes.
- Think about waste too: you can now buy lunchboxes that come with lidded containers that fit snugly within the external case. These can be reused rather than thrown away every day, dispensing with the need for excessive packaging, including cling film and foil.
- Make sure the lunchbox is easy to clean and that there are no nooks and crannies that are tricky to get at.

PRESENTATION

A little attention to detail can make a big difference to a lunchbox's appeal. Plastic tubs come in a range of shapes, sizes and colours and are perfect for dips, crudités, kebabs, salads, fruit, sandwiches and wraps. Avoid foods that are likely to break up or be damaged during transit (remember the mushy black banana that returns untouched!). Just including a range of different-coloured foods, especially fruit and vegetables, will add to its appeal.

BALANCING ACT

It may come as little surprise to learn that according to recent research the most popular items in a lunchbox are a sliced white bread sandwich with a filling of ham, cheese or chicken; crisps; a chocolate bar or biscuit; and a yogurt or cheese snack. While, there's nothing intrinsically wrong with any of these foods on an occasional basis, if a child eats them every day, they will not get the range of nutrients they need for good health. The key to a healthy packed lunch is nutritional balance and a wide variety of foods.

To make things easier, use the following guidelines as a template for your child's lunchbox. They show the importance of offering a variety of foods from the main food groups. By following these suggestions you can ensure your lunchbox provides the foods your child needs for health, development and well-being.

PUTTING IT INTO PRACTICE

A nutritionally balanced lunchbox should feature one or more items from each of the following food groups.

Fruit and veg

- Many of us struggle to get our kids to eat enough fruit and vegetables a day, yet the lunchbox provides the perfect opportunity to boost a child's consumption of fresh produce. Choose different types, which not only ensures your child gets a range of nutrients but also helps to avoid the boredom factor.

- Consider presenting fruit in different ways: in a fruit salad, compote, puréed, chopped, sliced, and so on. Look out for mini-packs of dried fruit, but do check the label first as some contain additives as well as added sugar and fat. Better still, make your own mixes, incorporating shredded coconut, nuts and seeds, which add vital nutrients.

- Children often prefer raw vegetables to cooked: cherry tomatoes or sticks of carrot, cucumber and pepper are popular, but you could also try slices of fennel, florets of broccoli and cauliflower, fresh peas, whole mangetouts, sugar snap peas, baby corn and salad leaves. Certain vegetables are best cooked, such as asparagus, beetroot, runner beans and green beans.

Dairy foods

- About half of adult bone density is laid down during adolescence, so it is important to provide good sources of calcium, such as dairy foods. Many of the cheeses for lunchboxes are of the processed variety – dippers, dunkers, strings and the like. Do check labels first but, better still, a healthier and cheaper option is to include a chunk of farmhouse cheese, preferably organic. Bear in mind that many cheeses are high in saturated fat so use in moderation or opt for lower-fat alternatives such as low-fat cream cheese, Quark, mozzarella, feta and Brie. (Non-dairy sources of calcium include green leafy vegetables, sardines, eggs, nuts, seeds and wholegrain cereals.)

- Look at the label on a fruit yogurt and you may find that it contains very little real fruit, if any, and then you have the additional undesirable sweeteners, sugar, colours and preservatives. To make your own fruit yogurt, simply purée or finely chop some fresh fruit and blend it with a cupful of thick and creamy natural bio yogurt, and a teaspoonful of clear honey or maple syrup if the fruit is a little tart. Yogurt, like fromage frais, is a first-class protein food, while bio versions contain "good" bacteria that benefit the digestive system. Adding a tablespoonful of toasted oats and seeds further boosts the vitamin and mineral content.

Protein

- Protein foods are great for staving off hunger-pangs and work in unison with carbohydrate foods, which provide long-term energy and help to boost concentration, memory and attention span. Use protein-rich foods in sandwich fillings, savoury dishes and salads, or to nibble on. Good examples are: lean, cooked chicken, turkey or beef; fish and prawns; eggs; nuts, nut butters and seeds; pulses and hummus; vegetarian sausages and nut cutlets; tofu.

- Children in particular need omega-3 essential fatty acids for their developing brains, eyes and nerves. Omega-3 has also been shown to improve mood and benefit those with dyslexia and attention deficit hyperactivity disorder. It is found in oily fish such as herring, salmon, trout, mackerel, sardines and tuna, which all make great sandwich fillings, pâtés, savoury dishes and salads.

Starchy carbs

- Whole grains are the body's main source of long-term energy and should be at the heart of a lunchbox. Bread is the obvious option and there are now so many different types to choose from: ditch white bread in favour of Granary or rye for healthy sandwiches; fill rolls, baps and bagels; use pitta breads as pockets or cut into strips for dipping; and use flat breads to wrap around fillings. Pastry cutters are a great way to make different-shaped sandwiches, adding extra interest for young eaters.

- Alternatively, try rice, noodles or potatoes. They all make a great base for a salad and hold up well to being transported. Combine cooked pasta or rice with diced red pepper, canned corn, fresh tomato and cubes of cheese, and lubricate with a spoonful of pesto and reduced-fat mayonnaise. Couscous and bulghur wheat are great with chopped tomato, cucumber, spring onion, olives and mint, then dressed with lemon juice and olive oil. Cooked noodles work with oriental-style dressings, such as a mix of soy sauce, sesame oil and fresh ginger.

Drinks

Most children don't drink enough fluids, especially while at school. Dehydration can affect concentration and intellectual performance, as well as the transportation of nutrients around the body. A 2-per-cent loss in body fluids, for example, can cause a 20-per-cent reduction in both physical and mental performance. Make sure you provide a bottle of water, diluted fresh fruit juice, or milk, and avoid carbonated and other sugary drinks. Most fruit drinks contain little in the way of fruit and lots of sugar, so opt for freshly squeezed instead and dilute with a little water.

If you find it difficult to get your child to drink water, fresh fruit smoothies and vegetable juices are a nutritious alternative and count as one portion out of the recommended servings of fruit and vegetables a day. There are plenty to choose from in the chiller cabinets of most supermarkets or they are simple to make at home: blend a banana with natural yogurt and a little milk for an energy-sustaining drink. Strawberries, nectarines, raspberries and mango are also good alternatives for a summery flavour. For a vegetable version, apple, carrot and beetroot is a colourful and tasty combination.

SHOPPING LIST

Ideally, lunchboxes should be appealing, inviting, "cool" enough to withstand scrutiny from peers, and never boring! If this sounds a tall order, then forward planning and organization make it that much easier. The first step is shopping – keep a list in the kitchen of what you need to buy for the week. Break the list down into various food types, including fresh foods with a limited shelf life, breads, chilled foods, frozen foods and storecupboard staples. Arming yourself with a list when shopping will also give you the strength to stand firm against pester power: "If it's not on the list, I'm not going to buy it!"

The following lists of foods make a helpful guide and a good starting point.

Fresh fruit and veg

These have a limited shelf life, so try to avoid wastage by not buying too much. Buy as fresh as possible and, if you can, opt for organic, seasonal fruit and vegetables. Make the most of local markets, farmer's markets and delivery boxes.

Choose from fruits such as kiwi fruit, melons, mangoes, pineapples, apples, grapes, citrus fruits, bananas, pears, nectarines, peaches, plums, strawberries, raspberries and blueberries. Also offer your child avocados, salad leaves, peppers, carrots, sweetcorn, broccoli, cauliflower, spring onions, tomatoes, beetroot, celery, cucumber, soya beans, green beans, potatoes, sweet potatoes, herbs, squash and sprouted seeds and beans.

Chilled foods

The following foods have a limited shelf life, so buy regularly in small amounts. These protein foods make a valuable contribution to a lunchbox, keeping hunger pangs at bay for the afternoon ahead. However, some are high in fat, so it's best to keep an eye on food labels and opt for lower-fat varieties. Nutritional chilled foods to choose from are: eggs, tofu, hummus, guacamole, dips, pâtés and spreads, deli meat, such as ham, salami, cooked chicken and so on, sausages, fish and shellfish, cheese, soup, mayonnaise, olives/sun-dried tomatoes, natural bio yogurt, fromage frais, rice pudding, fruit juice and smoothies.

Storecupboard

Most of these foods will keep for weeks or months and can readily form a central part of a lunchbox, so it's a good idea to keep a varied selection. Keep an eye on best-before and use-by dates and note that some products require chilling after opening.

The range is very wide, but here are some of the many foods that will form the backbone of your lunchbox ingredients:

KEEP IT SAFE

When preparing a lunchbox, pay special care to food safety and hygiene. Keep all foods, and especially those susceptible to food-poisoning bacteria, such as meat, poultry, fish, dairy, eggs, rice and other grains, well chilled. Pack in an insulated lunchbox with an ice pack or store in the fridge, if possible.

dried fruit (try to avoid those with added sugar and sulphur dioxide as they can exacerbate asthma), canned fruit, rice cakes, crackers, breadsticks, corn crackers, tortillas, couscous, bulghur wheat, barley, pasta, noodles, polenta, rice, canned beans and lentils, canned fish, nuts and seeds, flour, canned tomatoes and sweetcorn, pesto, herbs and spices, oats, nut butters, honey, high-fruit/low-sugar jam, pretzels, popcorn and low-sugar cereal bars.

Breads

Bread is most nutritious when made with wholemeal flour and also contains a higher amount of fibre. Try different varieties of bread to avoid the boredom factor and store a supply of bread in the freezer to avoid running out: wholemeal bread, bagels, pitta breads, focaccias, ciabattas, baps/rolls, flatbreads, baguettes, fruit bread, muffins, scones and currant buns.

Frozen foods

Frozen items can be a valuable asset when preparing a lunchbox. Freeze homemade soups and other prepared foods in single portions for future use. Frozen fruits and vegetables make a convenient standby and are often more nutritious than fresh, having been frozen soon after picking. Purées, compotes and sauces all freeze well. Choose vegetables, fruit, fish/shellfish, meat, soup, tarts, pies, bread, pizza, homemade burgers, falafel and potato cakes.

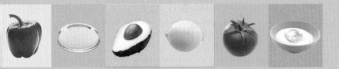

NIBBLES & DIPS

The varied recipes within this chapter will all add substance and variety with the minimum of effort or time – all positive attributes when making a lunchbox. They are also a way to get extra nutrition into children. Many children love to eat with their fingers, and a selection of vegetable sticks are perfect for dunking into healthy dips such as hummus, guacamole and tzatziki. While the Smoked Salmon Pâté and Smashed Bean & Carrot Spread can be dipped into as well, they are also delicious spread over pitta bread or crispbread. Presentation is a key factor in the success of a lunchbox, and "things on sticks", such as Mozzarella, Cherry Tomato & Basil or Salami, Cheese & Pineapple, will tempt even the fussiest of eaters.

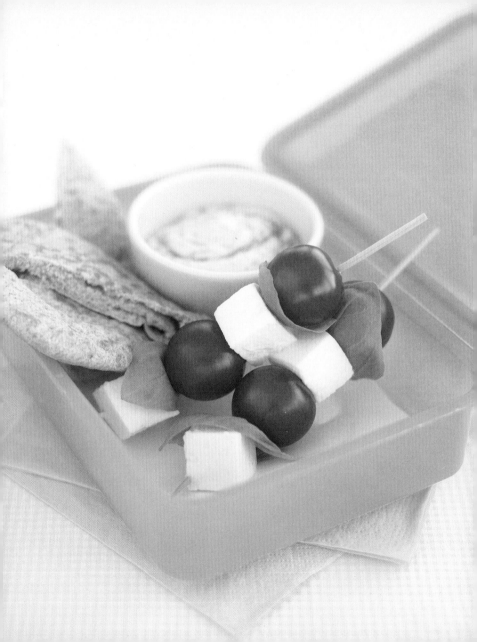

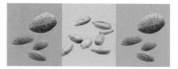

SERVES 4

PREPARATION + COOKING
5 + 10 minutes

STORAGE
Make in advance and keep in an airtight container for up to 1 week.

SERVE THIS WITH...
Pear & Ham Bundles
(see page 24)
Tabbouleh (see page 90)
fruit yogurt
fruit

HEALTH BENEFITS
Yes, nuts are high in fat but, on the whole, it is the healthy monounsaturated type. They're also rich in protein, calcium, iron, vitamin E, selenium and fibre. Seeds are good too, with pumpkin providing both omega-3 and omega-6 essential fatty acids.

soy-coated nuts & seeds

Shop-bought roasted nuts are generally deep-fried. Here the nuts and seeds are roasted without any fat, then lightly sprinkled with soy sauce. If nuts are a no-no, increase the seeds.

200g/7oz/scant 2 cups mixed unsalted nuts and seeds: peanuts (skins rubbed off), almonds, cashews, walnuts, hazelnuts, brazils, sunflower, hemp, pumpkin or linseeds
1–2 tsp soy sauce

1 Preheat the oven to 170°C/325°F/Gas 3. Place the nuts on a baking tray and roast for about 6 minutes. Add the seeds and roast for another 2–4 minutes until they smell toasted and are golden; watch carefully as they burn easily.
2 Remove from the oven and transfer to a bowl. Leave to cool slightly then drizzle with the soy sauce, turning the nuts and seeds with a spoon until they are coated.

Ⓥ Ⓧ Ⓧ Ⓧ Ⓟ

savoury spicy popcorn

Delicious as it is, popcorn doesn't have to be smothered in caramel or salt. For a healthier version, it's easy to make your own low-fat, sugar-free, salt-free alternative.

1 tbsp sunflower oil   1 tsp Cajun spice mix
70g/2½oz popping corn

1 Heat the oil in a saucepan, then add the popping corn in a single layer. Cover the pan with a lid and cook over a medium heat, shaking the pan frequently, until the corn has popped. Do not lift the lid until it has finished popping.
2 Transfer the popcorn to a large bowl and sprinkle the spice mix over the top. Turn the popcorn with a spoon until it is coated in the spices. Leave to cool.

SERVES 4

PREPARATION + COOKING
2 + 3 minutes

STORAGE
Make in advance and keep in an airtight container for up to 3 days.

SERVE THIS WITH…
Cool Dogs (see page 69)
salad
Strawberry Crunch Pot
 (see page 124)
fruit

HEALTH BENEFITS
Corn is one of the most nutritionally balanced carbohydrate foods and provides plenty of long-term energy.

003

Ⓥ ⊗ ⊗

cheesy celery sticks

A stick of celery makes a natural container for cream cheese or any type of pâté or thick dip. A halved and cored apple, pear or seeded cucumber would also work well.

SERVES 1

PREPARATION
5 minutes

STORAGE
Make on the day.

SERVE THIS WITH...
Roast Chicken & Avocado Focaccia (see page 67) Winter Fruit Salad (see page 122), puréed fruit yogurt

HEALTH BENEFITS
Celery was grown as a medicinal plant before it was even considered a food. Traditionally, it was used to treat nervousness, but it can also help to curb high blood pressure.

1 stick celery
1–2 tbsp low-fat cream cheese
   (flavour of choice)

1 Cut the celery in half or thirds, depending on its length.
2 Spread the cream cheese into the groove running down the pieces of celery.

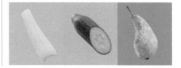

honey-sesame sausages

Buy the best-quality sausages you can, with a high meat content, preferably organic. Small cocktail sausages are easy for children to eat: serve in a pot or on some lettuce or cucumber.

2 tsp olive oil
1 tbsp clear honey
1 tsp Dijon mustard

12 good-quality
   cocktail sausages
1 tsp sesame seeds (optional)

1 Preheat the oven to 180°C/350°F/Gas 4. Mix together the oil, honey and mustard in a bowl. Add the sausages and turn to coat them in the mixture.
2 Arrange the sausages in a non-stick roasting tin and cook in the oven for about 12–14 minutes, turning occasionally, until almost cooked. Sprinkle the sesame seeds over, if using, and cook for another minute until the sausages are golden and cooked through. Leave to cool.

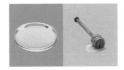

SERVES 2–4

PREPARATION + COOKING
5 + 15 minutes

STORAGE
Make in advance and keep in the fridge for up to 3 days. Keep chilled until ready to eat (see page 17).

SERVE THIS WITH...
Tzatziki (see page 34)
Cheese, Apple & Chutney Bap
  (see page 52)
natural yogurt with honey
fruit

HEALTH BENEFITS
Red meat is classed as a first-class protein, meaning that it provides all the amino acids required by the body for its growth and repair. It's also a good source of iron, and studies have found that children are often deficient in this mineral, which can influence behaviour and development.

pear & ham bundles

SERVES 1

PREPARATION
5 minutes

STORAGE
Make on the day. Keep chilled until ready to eat (see page 17).

SERVE THIS WITH...
Italian Flag Salad (see page 80)
chunk of bread
Apricot Cookie (see page 136)
fruit

HEALTH BENEFITS
Pears are one of the least allergenic of foods and are therefore excellent for children. Full of natural sweetness, pears also provide vitamin C, and fibre if the skin is left on.

Pear is a natural partner to Parma ham, as is melon, nectarine or peach. These bundles make a change from the obvious sandwich, and you could carry on the Italian theme with an Italian Flag Salad (see page 80) and a chunk of ciabatta. Alternatively, you could try wrapping the ham around some breadsticks.

1 ripe but not too soft pear, quartered and cored

squeeze of lemon juice
2 slices Parma ham, halved

1 Place the pear quarters on a plate, squeeze the lemon juice over them and turn until they are coated – this will help to prevent them browning.
2 Wrap one strip of Parma ham around each pear quarter.

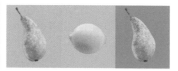

Ⓥ Ⓧ Ⓧ ⊘

mozzarella, cherry tomato & basil sticks

Attractive presentation can perk up a tired-looking lunchbox, and these colourful kebabs take only minutes to make. For young children, omit the sticks and serve in a small pot.

4 cherry tomatoes	Pesto dip:
4 basil leaves	2 tbsp low-fat natural
4 x 1cm/½in cubes	bio yogurt
mozzarella cheese	2 tsp green pesto

1 To make the dip, mix together the yogurt and pesto, then spoon into a small lidded pot.
2 Thread a cherry tomato on to a cocktail stick, followed by a basil leaf and a cube of mozzarella. Add a second tomato, basil leaf and cube of mozzarella, then assemble a second stick. Serve the sticks with the pesto dip.

SERVES 1

PREPARATION
10 minutes

STORAGE
Make the dip in advance and keep in the fridge for up to 1 week. Assemble the sticks on the day.

SERVE THIS WITH...
slices of wholemeal pitta bread
carrot sticks
Date & Pecan Brownie
(see page 133)
fruit

HEALTH BENEFITS
Mozzarella is relatively low in fat but still provides valuable amounts of bone-building calcium – vital for growing kids.

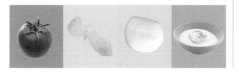

SERVES 1

PREPARATION + COOKING
10 + 6 minutes

STORAGE
Make in advance, and keep the dip in the fridge for up to 1 week and the chicken for up to 3 days. Keep chilled until ready to eat (see page 17).

SERVE THIS WITH…
carrot, cucumber and
   pepper sticks
wholemeal tortilla
Apricot Cookie (see page 136)
fruit

HEALTH BENEFITS
Chicken is an excellent source of low-fat protein and is a good source of selenium, which helps to support the immune system.

chicken strips with satay dip

Full of appetite-satisfying protein, these chicken sticks and peanut dip are fun to eat and easy to make. Tzatziki (page 34) or Tomato Salsa (page 30) can be served instead of the satay dip if peanuts are not allowed in your child's school.

1 tbsp olive oil
1 tsp paprika
140g/5oz skinless chicken
   breast, cut into 4–6 strips

Satay dip:
2 tbsp peanut butter

1 tsp olive oil
1 tsp tamari (wheat-free
   soy sauce)
½ tsp soft light brown sugar
1 tbsp reduced-fat coconut milk
   or mayonnaise

1 To make the satay dip, mix together all the ingredients with 1 tbsp hot water in a bowl until combined, then transfer to a lidded pot.
2 Put the oil in a shallow dish; add the paprika and then the chicken. Turn the chicken in the oil.
3 Heat a large frying pan and fry the chicken for about 2–3 minutes on each side until golden and cooked through. Leave to cool.
4 Serve the strips dipped into the satay sauce.

salami, cheese & pineapple sticks

A twist on the favourite cheese and pineapple combination. If you have fresh pineapple, so much the better, because it tends to be richer in vitamins than the canned version – although canned pineapple is more than adequate, especially if it is canned in natural juice.

4 thin slices salami
4 chunks pineapple

4 large bite-sized cubes Cheddar or other hard cheese

1 Fold a slice of salami in half then half again and thread on to a cocktail stick, followed by a chunk of pineapple, then a chunk of Cheddar.
2 Repeat to make four sticks.

MAKES 4

PREPARATION
5 minutes

STORAGE
Make the day before and keep in the fridge overnight. Keep chilled until ready to eat (see page 17).

SERVE THIS WITH…
Mixed Bean Salad (see page 82)
Custard Tartlet (see page 135)
fruit

HEALTH BENEFITS
Pineapple aids digestion, particularly that of protein foods, and has also been found to have anti-inflammatory properties.

*roasted red pepper hummus

HEALTH BENEFITS
Chickpeas are low in fat and a good source of both protein and carbohydrate. As an added bonus, they count as one of the recommended portions of fruit and vegetables we should eat each day.

Hummus is a versatile addition to a lunchbox. It makes a perfect dip with vegetable sticks or a sandwich filling. In addition, a spoonful can be added to soups. The roasted red pepper adds flavour and colour.

1 red pepper, seeded
  and quartered
3 tbsp extra-virgin olive oil,
  plus extra for drizzling
235g/8½oz/heaped 1½ cups
  canned no-salt, no-sugar
  chickpeas, drained
  and rinsed

2 cloves garlic, halved
1 heaped tbsp light tahini
  (sesame seed paste)
juice of ½ lemon
salt
freshly ground black pepper

SERVES 6

PREPARATION + COOKING
15 + 30 minutes

STORAGE
Make in advance and keep in the
fridge for up to 1 week.

1 Preheat the oven to 200°C/400°F/Gas 6. Put the pepper
quarters in a roasting tin with 1 tbsp of the oil. Toss the
pepper in the oil until coated, then roast for 25–30 minutes,
turning once, until the skin begins to blister and blacken.
2 Remove the pepper from the oven and leave until cool
enough to handle, then peel off the skin.
3 Put the pepper in a food processor or blender with the
chickpeas, garlic, tahini, lemon juice, 2 tbsp water and
the rest of the oil. Blend until the mixture forms a chunky,
creamy purée, occasionally scraping the mixture down
the sides of the processor or blender.
4 Transfer the hummus to a lidded pot. Season to taste
and drizzle a little extra olive oil over the top.

SERVE THIS WITH...
vegetable sticks, such as red
  pepper, cucumber, carrot, sugar
  snap peas and baby sweetcorn
seeded breadsticks
Ham & Egg Pie (see page 103)
fruit yogurt
fruit

**Garlic is
known for its
heart-protecting
properties and
is most potent
when raw.**

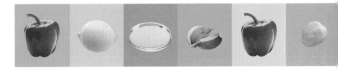

010

V

tortilla dippers with tomato salsa

SERVES 1 (SALSA FOR 4)

PREPARATION + COOKING
10 + 20 minutes

STORAGE
Make the salsa in advance and keep in the fridge for up to 3 days or freeze for up to 1 month. Cook the tortilla wedges on the day.

SERVE THIS WITH...
Honey-sesame Sausages (see page 23)
Apple Coleslaw (see page 76)
muffin
fruit

HEALTH BENEFITS
Tomatoes contain antioxidants, including significant amounts of vitamins E and C and beta-carotene, which have a protective effect on the body. Canned tomatoes have similar nutritional values to fresh.

Crispy tortillas are delicious dunked into this rich tomato salsa or some Roasted Red Pepper Hummus (see page 28), Creamy Guacamole (see page 31) or Tzatziki (see page 34).

1 wholemeal tortilla
1 tsp olive oil

Tomato salsa:
2 tbsp olive oil
2 cloves garlic, crushed

350ml/12fl oz/1½ cups passata (sieved tomatoes)
1 tbsp sun-dried tomato paste
½ tsp sugar
2 tomatoes, seeded and cut into small pieces (optional)

1 To make the tomato salsa, heat the oil in a saucepan. Fry the garlic for 1 minute, stirring to prevent it burning. Add the passata, tomato paste and sugar, then bring to the boil. Reduce the heat to low, half-cover the pan with a lid and simmer for 15 minutes. Stir the sauce occasionally to prevent it sticking to the bottom of the pan. Leave to cool then stir in the fresh tomatoes, if using.
2 Cut the tortilla in half and then into three or four wedges depending on its size. Heat the oil in a frying pan and fry the wedges in batches for about 2 minutes on each side until golden and crisp. When cool, pack with the salsa.

Ⓥ Ⓧ Ⓧ Ⓐ Ⓞ

creamy guacamole

Crispy raw vegetables are often more acceptable to children than cooked, and even the most unlikely of veg are good served in this way. Try extending the choice from peppers, carrots and cucumbers to florets of cauliflower, broccoli, sugar snap peas, mangetout and baby corn. If time allows, make the guacamole on the day of serving because it is best as fresh as possible.

1 ripe avocado, halved and
   stone removed
1 clove garlic, crushed
juice of ½ small lemon or
   juice of 1 lime

1 tbsp mayonnaise
1 tbsp finely chopped fresh
   coriander (optional)
salt
freshly ground black pepper

1 Use a spoon to scoop the avocado out of its skin into a bowl. Stir in the garlic, lemon or lime juice and mayonnaise and mash using a fork to achieve the consistency you want.
2 Stir in the coriander, if using, and season to taste.

SERVES 4

PREPARATION
10 minutes

STORAGE
Make the day before and keep in the fridge overnight, or make on the day.

SERVE THIS WITH....
vegetable sticks, such as
   mangetout, baby sweetcorn
   and broccoli florets
Falafel & Hummus Lavash
   (see page 68), replacing the
   hummus
Carrot Cake (see page 134)
fruit

HEALTH BENEFITS
Avocados have recently been found to be a good source of lutein, which protects the eyes against disease such as cataracts and age-related degeneration.

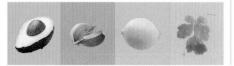

SERVES 4–6

PREPARATION + COOKING
15 + 40 minutes

STORAGE
Make in advance and keep in the fridge for up to 5 days.

SERVE THIS WITH...
breadsticks or pitta bread slices
carrot, cucumber, celery and/or
  sweet pepper sticks
Spicy Sweet Potatoes
  (see page 95)
fruit

HEALTH BENEFITS
Look for bright, shiny, firm aubergines, which will be a richer source of vitamins B and C than those that are past their best.

roasted aubergine dip

If your child is not keen on aubergine, then why not try it in this slightly spicy, smoky, garlicky dip? It's good spread on pitta bread or dipped into with breadsticks and vegetable sticks.

1 large aubergine	1 tsp ground coriander
2 cloves garlic	2 tbsp extra-virgin olive oil
1 tbsp light tahini	juice of ½ lemon
(sesame seed paste)	salt
1 tsp ground cumin	freshly ground black pepper

1 Preheat the oven to 200°C/400°F/Gas 6. Prick the aubergine all over with a fork, then place in a roasting tin. Roast for about 40 minutes, until the inside of the aubergine is very soft.

2 Leave to cool slightly, then halve the aubergine lengthways and scoop out the flesh with a spoon into a food processor or blender. Add the garlic, tahini, spices, olive oil and lemon juice. Process until smooth and creamy. Season to taste.

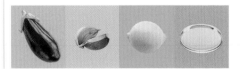

smashed bean & carrot spread

Butter beans have a bit of an image problem, but if combined with stronger flavours such as spices they make a great base for a spread.

1 carrot, sliced
2 tbsp extra-virgin olive oil
2 cloves garlic, crushed
1 tsp ground cumin
¼ tsp ground cinnamon
1 tsp ground coriander

2 pinches chilli powder
200g/7oz/1½ cups canned butter
   beans, drained and rinsed
juice of 1 lemon
salt
freshly ground black pepper

1 Steam the carrot until tender. Meanwhile, heat the oil in a saucepan and fry the garlic and spices for 1 minute. Add the beans, lemon juice and 2–3 tbsp water, then heat gently, stirring.
2 Put the carrot in a food processor or blender with the bean mixture. Process until smooth, adding a little extra water if necessary, then season to taste.

SERVES 4–6

PREPARATION + COOKING
10 + 5 minutes

STORAGE
Make in advance and keep in the fridge for up to 5 days.

TRY THIS WITH…
pitta bread or flatbread
Melon & Halloumi Salad
   (see page 78)
cookie

HEALTH BENEFITS
Canned beans are not only convenient but also a good source of low-fat protein, fibre, iron, magnesium and B vitamins.

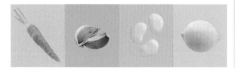

⓿❽❽

tzatziki

This Greek dip is traditionally made using yogurt and cucumber, flavoured with mint and served with pitta bread. This version uses low-fat natural bio yogurt and finely grated courgette, which contains less water than cucumber and so holds together better.

SERVES 2

PREPARATION
10 minutes

STORAGE
Make in advance and keep in the fridge for up to 3 days.

SERVE THIS WITH...
wholemeal pitta bread
Falafel (see page 104)
Apple Flapjack (see page 126)
fruit

HEALTH BENEFITS
Studies show that certain cultures in yogurt may help to boost immunity, protect against infection and support the digestive system by increasing the amount of "friendly" bacteria in the gut.

4 tbsp low-fat natural
   bio yogurt
5cm/2in piece courgette,
   finely grated

1 small clove garlic, crushed
2 tbsp finely chopped mint
salt
freshly ground black pepper

1 Mix together the yogurt, courgette, garlic and mint in a lidded pot or bowl.
2 Season to taste.

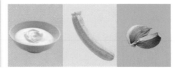

smoked salmon pâté

Children are recommended to eat at least one portion of oily fish a week, and this creamy smoked salmon pâté is ideal and simple to prepare. You could use smoked mackerel or smoked trout as an alternative.

175g/6oz smoked salmon pieces
juice of ½ lemon, or to taste

100g/3½oz low-fat cream cheese
½ tsp paprika
freshly ground black pepper

1 Put the salmon, lemon juice, cream cheese and paprika into a blender or food processor. Process until smooth and creamy. Season with pepper to taste.
2 Transfer to a bowl, cover and put in the fridge.

SERVES ABOUT 6

PREPARATION
10 minutes

STORAGE
Make in advance and keep in the fridge for up to 3 days. Keep chilled until ready to eat (see page 17).

SERVE THIS WITH...
Oat Biscuits (see page 137)
cherry tomatoes and cucumber sticks
Carrot Cake (see page 134)
fruit

HEALTH BENEFITS
Smoked salmon is a rich source of omega-3 essential fatty acids, which benefit a child's developing brain, eyes and nervous system.

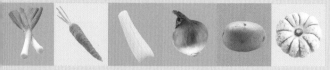

SOUPS

Soup makes a fantastic addition to a lunchbox – wholesome, warming, versatile and nutritious. The colder winter months can put parents off packed lunches in favour of a warm school meal, but many lunchboxes now come with a small unbreakable flask, allowing soup to be taken to school. Soups keep well and are ideal for making in advance: either chill or freeze in portions and reheat on the day. Chunky homemade vegetable, bean, pasta or noodle soups make a complete meal, providing both protein and carbohydrates. Puréed soups are great for children who dislike "bits" or won't eat vegetables, since the smooth texture disguises the ingredients. To make a nutritious and balanced lunch, just add some bread and a chunk of cheese or slice of cold meat.

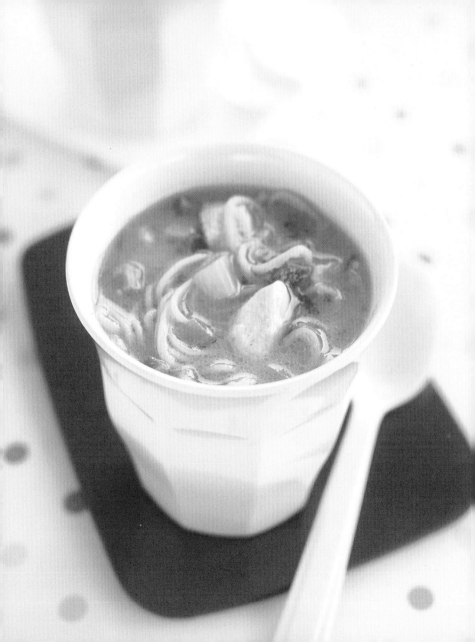

SERVES 4

PREPARATION + COOKING
15 + 35 minutes

STORAGE
Make in advance and keep in the fridge for up to 3 days or freeze in single portions.

SERVE THIS WITH...
onion bagel
Strawberry Crunch Pot
  (see page 124)
dried apricots

HEALTH BENEFITS
Tomatoes get their colour from a natural plant compound called lycopene, which is best absorbed by the body when tomatoes are cooked. Lycopene has been found to protect us from some cancers and heart disease.

creamy tomato & lentil soup

Tomato is many children's favourite soup. This version contains a nutritional boost, thanks to the lentils, which become hidden when cooked.

85g/3oz/$\frac{1}{3}$ cup split red lentils
1 tbsp olive oil
1 large onion, chopped
1 carrot, chopped
400ml/14fl oz/1$\frac{2}{3}$ cups passata
  (sieved tomatoes)

900ml/1$\frac{1}{2}$ pints/3$\frac{3}{4}$ cups
  gluten-free vegetable stock
1 bay leaf
4 tbsp reduced-fat crème fraîche
salt
freshly ground black pepper

1 Rinse the lentils, put in a saucepan, cover with water and bring to the boil. Reduce the heat and simmer, half-covered, for 15 minutes until tender. Drain and set aside.

2 Meanwhile, heat the oil in a large saucepan. Add the onion and fry, half-covered, for 7 minutes, then add the carrot. Fry the vegetables, half-covered, for another 3 minutes, stirring occasionally.

3 Add the passata, stock, cooked lentils and bay leaf. Bring to the boil, then reduce the heat and simmer, part-covered, for 20 minutes until the vegetables are tender.

4 Purée in a blender or using a hand-held blender. Stir in the crème fraîche, season to taste and heat through gently.

V

green giant soup

Petits pois (young peas) have a delicate, sweet flavour and tender outer skin that work well in this vibrantly coloured green soup.

1 tbsp olive oil
1 large leek, finely chopped
1 stick celery, thinly sliced
1 bay leaf
2 large sprigs mint (optional)
2 potatoes, peeled and cubed

1.2 litres/2 pints/5 cups
   gluten-free vegetable stock
250g/9oz/heaped 2 cups frozen
   petits pois
120ml/4fl oz/½ cup milk
   (optional)

1 Heat the oil in a large saucepan and fry the leek for 5 minutes until softened. Add the celery, bay leaf, mint, if using, and potatoes and cook, half-covered, for 3 minutes.
2 Pour in the stock and bring to the boil. Reduce the heat, half-cover and simmer for 20 minutes. Add the peas and cook for another 5 minutes until the vegetables are tender.
3 Purée in a blender or using a hand-held blender. Return to the pan and stir in the milk, if using, or more stock and heat through gently. Season to taste.

SERVES 4

PREPARATION + COOKING
10 + 35 minutes

STORAGE
Make in advance and keep in the fridge for up to 3 days or freeze in single portions.

SERVE THIS WITH...
strips of crispy grilled bacon to dip in or to crush and sprinkle over the top
Cheese Scones (see page 138)
fruit

HEALTH BENEFITS
Little nuggets of goodness, frozen peas are often richer in nutrients than fresh ones. A good source of protein and fibre, peas also provide iron, vitamins C and B and folate.

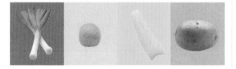

V

sweetcorn chowder

If sweetcorn is in season, use the corn from 3–4 fresh cobs; if not, use canned.

SERVES 4

PREPARATION + COOKING
10 + 35 minutes

STORAGE
Make in advance and keep in the fridge for up to 3 days or freeze in single portions.

SERVE THIS WITH…
crusty roll
chunk of cheese or ham
Date & Pecan Brownie
 (see page 133)
fruit

HEALTH BENEFITS
Sweetcorn is a rich source of nutrients, such as energy-giving carbohydrates, fibre, potassium, iron and vitamins A, B and C.

1 tbsp sunflower oil
1 large onion, chopped
1 carrot, chopped
2 potatoes, peeled and cubed
3–4 sweetcorn cobs, corn
 sliced off (optional)
1 bay leaf

900ml/1½ pints/3¾ cups
 gluten-free vegetable stock
400g/14oz can no-salt, no-sugar
 sweetcorn, drained (optional)
300ml/10fl oz/1¼ cups milk
salt
freshly ground black pepper

1 Heat the oil in a large saucepan and fry the onion for 7 minutes, half-covered, until softened. Add the carrot, potatoes, fresh corn (if using) and bay leaf and cook, half-covered, for another 3 minutes.

2 Pour in the stock, bring to the boil, reduce the heat and simmer for 10 minutes. Add the canned sweetcorn (if using) and simmer for a further 15 minutes, stirring occasionally.

3 Pour in the milk, gently heat through, then season to taste. Serve chunky, semi-chunky or smooth, as wanted.

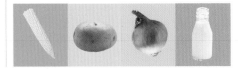

Ⓥ Ⓧ Ⓧ Ⓧ Ⓓ

spicy carrot & lentil soup

This lightly spiced soup provides an impressive collection of nutrients. Red lentils are perfect for thickening soups because they eventually break down during cooking into a comforting purée.

1 tbsp sunflower oil
1 large onion, chopped
1 stick celery, finely chopped
4 carrots, thinly sliced
140g/5oz/²/₃ cup split
    red lentils

1 tsp ground cumin
1 tbsp mild curry powder
1.2 litres/2 pints/5 cups
    gluten-free vegetable stock
salt
freshly ground black pepper

1 Heat the oil in a large saucepan and fry the onion over a medium-low heat for 7 minutes, half-covered, until softened. Add the celery and carrots and cook for another 3 minutes. Rinse the lentils.

2 Stir in the spices and lentils and cook, stirring, for 1 minute, then pour in the stock. Bring to the boil then reduce the heat and simmer, half-covered, for 35 minutes until the lentils are very soft and mushy. Occasionally skim off any foam created by the lentils during cooking.

3 Purée in a blender or using a hand-held blender. Season to taste.

SERVES 4

PREPARATION + COOKING
15 + 50 minutes

STORAGE
Make in advance and keep in the fridge for up to 3 days or freeze in single portions.

SERVE THIS WITH...
wholemeal pitta bread
Winter Fruit Salad (see page 122)

HEALTH BENEFITS
Sometimes known as Egyptian lentils, split red lentils are an excellent low-fat protein food, full of immune-supporting antioxidants.

Ⓥ Ⓧ Ⓧ Ⓧ

hallowe'en soup

Pumpkin or squash makes a thick, creamy soup with a touch of sweetness that goes down well with children.

SERVES 4

PREPARATION + COOKING
15 + 30 minutes

STORAGE
Make in advance and keep in the fridge for up to 3 days or freeze in single portions.

SERVE THIS WITH...
wholemeal bread
chunk of cheese or slices of ham
Banana & Blueberry Muffin
(see page 132)
fruit

HEALTH BENEFITS
The orange flesh of the pumpkin or squash provides plentiful amounts of beta-carotene as well as vitamins B, C and E, magnesium and potassium. Our bodies are more able to make the most of beta-carotene when it is cooked with a little oil.

1 tbsp olive oil
1 onion, chopped
1 carrot
1 stick celery, chopped
350g/12oz peeled pumpkin or
    butternut squash,
    cut into chunks
1 bay leaf (optional)

1 tsp dried mixed herbs
    (optional)
1 tbsp curry powder (optional)
2 sprigs rosemary
1.2 litres/2 pints/5 cups
    gluten-free vegetable stock
salt
freshly ground black pepper

1 Heat the oil in a large saucepan and fry the onion for 7 minutes, then add the carrot, celery and pumpkin or squash. Half-cover the pan and cook for another 3 minutes.
2 Add the herbs (or curry powder for a spicy soup) and stock. Bring to the boil, then reduce the heat and simmer, half-covered, for 20 minutes until the vegetables are tender.
3 Remove the bay leaf and rosemary. Purée in a blender or using a hand-held blender. Season to taste.

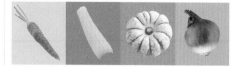

Ⓥ Ⓡ Ⓞ ⓓ

miso & tofu broth

Look out for sachets of instant miso in supermarkets and health-food stores. They simply need the addition of hot water to make a simple savoury stock and are an excellent base for a speedy Japanese-style soup.

55g/2oz fine egg noodles
1 sachet instant miso
   soup powder
½ carrot, cut into very thin strips
1 spring onion, cut into
   thin strips
1 tsp soy sauce
1 tsp toasted sesame seeds

finger-nail piece fresh ginger,
   peeled and cut into
   thin strips
4 x 1cm/½in cubes soft tofu
sprinkling of nori flakes
   (optional)
pinch of dried chilli flakes
   (optional)

1 Cook the noodles following the packet instructions; drain.
2 Rehydrate the instant miso soup powder in a saucepan, following the packet instructions.
3 Add the cooked noodles, carrot, spring onion, soy sauce, sesame seeds, ginger, tofu, nori flakes and chilli, if using, and heat through for 1 minute.

SERVES 1

PREPARATION + COOKING
10 + 5 minutes

STORAGE
Make on the day.

SERVE THIS WITH...
Summer Pudding (see page 130)
fruit

HEALTH BENEFITS
Miso, which is made from a combination of cooked soya beans, rice, wheat or barley that is left to ferment, is said to help eliminate toxins from the body.

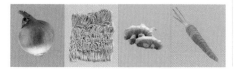

(V) (⊠)

chunky
italian soup

HEALTH BENEFITS
There's an element of truth in the adage that carrots help you see in the dark. Research has shown that eating just one carrot a day can help improve night vision; this is owing to its significant beta-carotene content. Chickpeas are high in zinc.

This nutritionally balanced soup contains carbohydrate, protein, fibre, vitamins and minerals – in fact, it's a complete meal in itself that will keep energy levels well sustained for the afternoon ahead.

55g/2oz/½ cup small pasta
   shapes such as conchigliette
   (small shells)
1 tbsp olive oil
1 onion, chopped
1 stick celery, chopped
1 large carrot, diced
1 tsp dried oregano

2 bay leaves
1.2 litres/2 pints/5 cups
   vegetable stock
100ml/3½fl oz/scant ½ cup
   passata (sieved tomatoes)
100g/3½oz/scant 1 cup canned
   no-salt, no-sugar chickpeas,
   drained and rinsed

SERVES 4–6

PREPARATION + COOKING
15 + 30 minutes

STORAGE
Make in advance and keep in the
fridge for up to 3 days or freeze
in single portions.

SERVE THIS WITH...
chunk of cheese or slices of ham
 or sausage
Apple Flapjack (see page 126)
fruit

1 Cook the pasta following the instructions on the packet
until al dente; drain and rinse under cold running water.
2 Meanwhile, put the oil in a large saucepan and add the
onion. Half-cover the pan and sauté the onion for 7 minutes,
stirring occasionally. Add the celery, carrot and herbs and
sauté for another 3 minutes.
3 Pour in the stock and passata and add the chickpeas.
Bring to the boil, then reduce the heat and simmer,
half-covered, for 15 minutes. Add the pasta, stir and cook
for another 5 minutes.

> **Chickpeas are low
> in fat and high in
> fibre. They are
> equally delicious
> hot or cold, and
> are very versatile.**

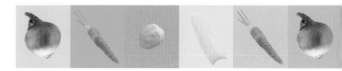

023

chicken noodle soup

Nurturing and sustaining, this is a great soup for a cold winter's day. For a vegetarian soup use vegetable stock and Quorn or extra veg.

SERVES 4

PREPARATION + COOKING
15 + 35 minutes

STORAGE
Make in advance and keep in the fridge for up to 3 days or freeze in single portions (unless the chicken was frozen).

SERVE THIS WITH...
Carrot Cake (see page 134)
fruit

HEALTH BENEFITS
A useful low-fat (as long as it is skinless) source of protein, chicken also provides selenium. This mineral is often missing in the diet and is a valuable immunity-boosting antioxidant.

55g/2oz/½ cup fine egg noodles
1 tbsp olive oil
1 onion, finely chopped
1 stick celery, finely chopped
1 carrot, diced
1 bay leaf
200g/7oz skinless chicken
    breast, cut into
    bite-sized pieces

1.2 litres/2 pints/5 cups
    chicken stock
2 tbsp reduced-fat
    crème fraîche
1 tbsp chopped flat-leaf parsley
    (optional)
salt
freshly ground black pepper

1 Cook the noodles following the packet instructions until al dente; drain and rinse under cold running water.
2 Meanwhile, put the oil in a large saucepan and add the onion. Half-cover the pan and sauté the onion for 7 minutes, stirring occasionally. Add the celery, carrot and bay leaf and sauté for another 3 minutes.
3 Add the chicken and sauté for 3–4 minutes, turning occasionally, until the chicken is golden all over.
4 Pour in the stock and bring to the boil, then reduce the heat and simmer for 20 minutes until the chicken is cooked. Stir in the crème fraîche and cooked noodles and warm through. Season and add the parsley, if using.

ham & barley broth

A complete meal in a pot – this soup contains carbohydrate (barley) and protein (pancetta), plus a healthy amount of vegetables. Vegetarians can omit the ham and serve cheese on the side.

100g/3½oz pearl barley
1 tbsp olive oil
1 large leek, finely sliced
1 large carrot, finely diced
85g/3oz pancetta or lean
    smoky bacon, diced
1 bay leaf
1 tsp dried mixed herbs
1.2 litres/2 pints/5 cups
    wheat-free vegetable stock
salt
freshly ground black pepper

1 Soak the barley in cold water for about 2 hours – this will help to speed up the cooking time. Drain and rinse.
2 Heat the olive oil in a large saucepan and fry the leek for 5 minutes, then add the carrot, pancetta or bacon and barley and cook for another 2 minutes.
3 Add the herbs and stock and bring to the boil. Reduce the heat and simmer, half-covered, for 40–45 minutes, stirring occasionally, until the barley is tender. Season to taste.

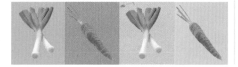

SERVES 4

PREPARATION + COOKING
10 + 55 minutes + soaking

STORAGE
Make in advance and keep in the fridge for up to 3 days or freeze in single portions.

SERVE THIS WITH...
chunk of cheese
Roasted Red Pepper Hummus
  (see page 28)
breadsticks
cereal bar
fruit

HEALTH BENEFITS
Believed to be the oldest cultivated grain, barley contains fibre, iron, calcium and B vitamins. In traditional medicine, barley is thought to boost physical strength.

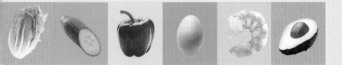

SANDWICHES & WRAPS

With such an abundance of different breads to choose from, there is no need to stick to the same type every day. Experiment with various varieties such as pitta breads, flatbreads, bagels, rolls, ciabatta and baguettes, and breads made with different types of flour, such as sourdough and Granary. Cut sliced bread into interesting shapes using pastry cutters or roll it to create spirals. Wraps are a great idea for lunchboxes: cover soft flour tortilla wraps with all manner of fillings, then roll them up. Or why not try using rice paper wraps, lettuce leaves or even an omelette as a wrap – an altogether more interesting variation on bread?

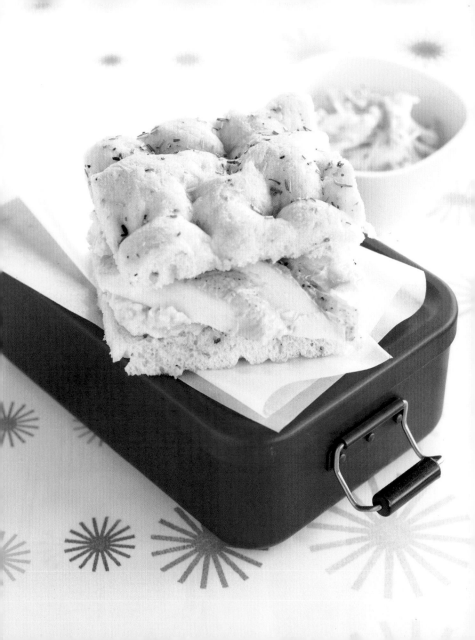

SERVES ABOUT 8

PREPARATION + COOKING
15 + 5 minutes

STORAGE
Make the nut butter in advance
and keep in the fridge for up to
2 weeks. Assemble on the day.

SERVE THIS WITH...
Cheesy Celery Sticks
  (see page 22)
carrot sticks
Chewy Date Bar (see page 127)
fruit

HEALTH BENEFITS
Cashew nuts are high in iron,
zinc, magnesium, selenium
and B vitamins – a great
immune-boosting combination.

nut butter & banana bagel

The beauty of home-made nut butter is that
you can choose your favourite combination of
nuts and use no additives. If you can't find a
cold-pressed oil that includes a blend of omega
fats, use sunflower or rapeseed oil instead.

1 sesame seed bagel
½ small banana, thinly sliced

Nut butter:
55g/2oz/½ cup unsalted
  cashew nuts

55g/2oz/½ cup unsalted
  peanuts
4–5 tbsp omega-blend or
  sunflower or rapeseed oil
½ tsp salt

1 Lightly toast the nuts in a dry frying pan over a
medium-low heat for 4–5 minutes, turning regularly, until
the nuts smell slightly toasted and are a light golden colour.
2 Leave the nuts to cool and rub off the brown papery
skin covering the peanuts, if necessary. Put the nuts, oil
and salt in a food processor and blend to a coarse paste.
Place the nut butter in a lidded jar in the fridge.
3 Cut the bagel in half and spread the nut butter over one
half. Arrange the slices of banana on top and cover with
the other bagel half.

(V)

cream cheese & date bagel

Low-fat cream cheese is a perfect base for many different flavourings, both sweet and savoury. Its smooth, creamy texture also means that there is no need for butter.

2 ready-to-eat dried dates   1 cinnamon bagel
1 tbsp low-fat cream cheese

1 Snip the dates into small pieces using scissors. Mix the dates into the cream cheese.
2 Cut the bagel in half and spread the date and cream cheese filling in the middle.

SERVES 1

PREPARATION
5 minutes

STORAGE
Make on the day.

SERVE THIS WITH...
Apple Coleslaw (see page 76)
cookie
fruit

HEALTH BENEFITS
Dates are a rich source of iron, which is essential for the formation of red blood cells and so needed for circulation.

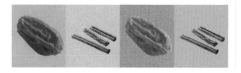

V ⊘

cheese, apple & chutney bap

Cheddar cheese and apple are a great combo. The homemade fresh fruity chutney is delicious, but you could use a little mayonnaise instead.

SERVES 1

PREPARATION + COOKING
15 + 30 minutes

STORAGE
Make the chutney in advance and keep in an airtight jar in the fridge for up to 2 weeks. Assemble on the day.

SERVE THIS WITH...
Super Salad (see page 81)
cereal bar
fruit

HEALTH BENEFITS
Although hard cheeses such as Cheddar tend to be higher in fat than soft cheeses, they are a better source of easily absorbable calcium and zinc. Using a mature cheese rather than a mild one means you'll need less cheese to obtain the same depth of flavour.

2–3 tbsp grated mature
    Cheddar cheese
½ small apple, cored
    and grated
1 seeded wholemeal bap

Chutney:
4 tomatoes, roughly chopped
1 large apple, peeled, cored
    and roughly chopped
1 onion, grated
5 tbsp white wine vinegar
55g/2oz/¼ cup sugar

1 Put all the chutney ingredients in a saucepan. Bring to the boil, then reduce the heat, cover and simmer for 5 minutes. Uncover the pan, then cook for a further 20 minutes. Leave to cool and spoon into a lidded jar.
2 Mix together the cheese, apple and 2 tsp chutney. Cut the bap in half and add the filling.

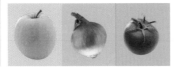

(V) (⏵)

mystery roll

Children will love this hollowed-out crusty roll with its hidden filling. This typical Provençal "sandwich", otherwise known as *pan bagnat*, is best made the day before to allow the flavours to mingle. You could use tuna, chicken or roasted vegetables instead of the cheese.

1 crusty roll
olive oil, for brushing
1–2 tbsp pesto
1 small clove garlic, crushed
  (optional)

4 slices mozzarella cheese
1 tomato, seeded and sliced
small handful of baby
  spinach leaves

1 Slice off the top of the roll to make a lid and pull out the soft inside, leaving the crust intact. Lightly brush the inside of the roll with olive oil.

2 Put the bread in a food processor and pulse until you have breadcrumbs. Transfer to a bowl and stir in sufficient pesto to flavour the breadcrumbs without making them soggy, and the garlic, if using.

3 Spoon a layer of the breadcrumbs into the roll. Add a layer of mozzarella, tomato and spinach followed by the rest of the breadcrumbs and the remaining mozzarella, tomato and spinach. Place the lid on top and wrap tightly. Press down lightly.

SERVES 1

PREPARATION
15 minutes

STORAGE
Make the day before and keep in the fridge overnight.

SERVE THIS WITH...
Savoury Spicy Popcorn
  (see page 21)
celery sticks
Cinnamon-spiced Apples
  (see page 120)

HEALTH BENEFITS
Spinach is one of the most nutritious of salad leaves and has a milder, less bitter flavour when uncooked, which also means it is richer in vitamins C and B. It also provides significant amounts of the eye-protecting antioxidant lutein.

Ⓥ ☺

bbq tofu baguette

The sweet, sticky marinade gives the tofu a rich, golden colour and smoky BBQ taste. Griddling the tofu also enhances its BBQ flavour, although you could fry it in a little oil or roast in the oven for 20 minutes instead.

SERVES 1 (TOFU SERVES 2)

PREPARATION + COOKING
10 + 8 minutes + marinating

STORAGE
Prepare and cook the tofu in advance and keep chilled for up to 3 days. Assemble on the day.

SERVE THIS WITH...
cucumber and celery sticks
Strawberry Crunch Pot
  (see page 124)
fruit

HEALTH BENEFITS
Tofu is the richest non-dairy source of calcium – in fact, a 100g/3½oz serving provides about half the daily allowance of calcium required by the 11–24 years age group.

olive oil, for brushing
125g/4½oz firm tofu, patted dry
  and cut into 4 long slices
1 small baguette
1 lettuce leaf, shredded
1 tomato, seeded and
  thinly sliced

Marinade:
1 tbsp clear honey or
  sweet chilli sauce
1 tbsp tomato ketchup
1 tbsp soy sauce
¼ tsp smoked paprika
  (optional)

1 In a shallow dish, mix together the ingredients for the marinade. Place the tofu slices in the dish with the marinade. Spoon the marinade over the tofu so it is well coated. Leave to marinate for at least 1 hour or overnight.
2 Generously brush a griddle pan with olive oil, then heat until hot. Carefully put the tofu slices in the pan and cook for 4 minutes on each side until golden, occasionally spooning over more of the marinade.
3 Slice the baguette lengthways and open it out. Place two of the tofu slices in the baguette and top with the lettuce and tomato. Close up the baguette and press down lightly.

egg & bacon roll

You can't beat egg and bacon as a flavour combination, but this version also benefits from the tomato and super-healthy alfalfa sprouts.

1 rasher bacon
1 free-range egg
1 ciabatta roll

½ tomato, seeded
few alfalfa sprouts or cress
freshly ground black pepper

1 Preheat the grill to medium-high and line the grill pan with foil. Grill the bacon until crisp, then leave to cool.
2 Meanwhile, boil the egg for about 6 minutes until the yolk is still very slightly runny. Hold the egg under cold running water until it is cool enough to handle.
3 Peel the egg, place in a bowl and roughly chop. Cut the bacon into small pieces and stir into the egg. Season.
4 Cut the ciabatta roll in half. Squeeze the tomato half and rub it into one half of the ciabatta. Spoon the egg and bacon mixture over the top and sprinkle with a few alfalfa sprouts or cress. Put the other half of the ciabatta on top.

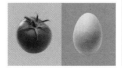

SERVES 1

PREPARATION + COOKING
10 + 7 minutes

STORAGE
Make the filling the day before and keep in the fridge overnight. Assemble on the day. Keep chilled until ready to eat (see page 17).

SERVE THIS WITH...
Creamy Guacamole (see page 31) and crudités
Apple Flapjack (see page 126)
fruit

HEALTH BENEFITS
Combining foods can improve the absorption of nutrients. The iron uptake from the eggs and bacon can be enhanced by eating them with vitamin C-rich foods such as tomatoes and alfalfa. A glass of fresh orange juice will also be of benefit.

herrings on rye

This is best assembled at the time of eating, which means it's probably more suitable for older children. Store the herrings in a lidded pot, then spoon them on to slices of rye bread. Herrings come in various marinades, including mustard, red onion and sweet vinegar, so choose what you think will go down the best.

SERVES 1

PREPARATION
5 minutes

STORAGE
Make on the day. Keep chilled until ready to eat (see page 17).

SERVE THIS WITH...
sliced beetroot
vegetable crisps
Banana & Blueberry Muffin
  (see page 132)
fruit

HEALTH BENEFITS
Herring is part of the oily fish family. There are literally hundreds of pieces of research that show the benefits of eating oily fish, from reducing blood pressure and cholesterol to improving brain power and concentration.

**low-fat cream cheese,
  for spreading**

**2 slices rye bread
6 slices marinated herring**

1 Spread the cream cheese over each slice of rye bread and sandwich with the cheesy sides in the middle.
2 Put the herrings in a pot with a lid. To eat, fork the herrings on to the bread or eat them separately straight from the pot, if that is easier.

sardines & tomato on brown

Canned sardines are not only a convenient storecupboard essential; they're also healthy, economical and versatile. If your child is anti-fish, try experimenting with the different flavour options available.

120g/4oz can sardines in olive
   oil, drained
1 tomato, seeded and
   finely chopped

1 tsp mayonnaise
½ tsp grain or mild mustard
2 slices wholemeal bread
   (toasted if preferred)

1 Put the sardines in a bowl and mash with a fork. Add the tomato and mix with the sardines.

2 Mix together the mayonnaise and mustard and spread over one slice of bread. Spoon on the sardines and tomato, and place the other slice of bread on top. Cut into triangles.

SERVES 1

PREPARATION
10 minutes

STORAGE
Make on the day. Keep chilled until ready to eat (see page 17).

SERVE THIS WITH...
carrot sticks
Soy-coated Nuts & Seeds
  (see page 20)
Summer Fruit Salad
  (see page 121)

HEALTH BENEFITS
All canned oily fish provide omega-3 fatty acids, although canned tuna has negligible amounts. Canned sardines have very soft bones that are barely distinguishable but are an excellent source of calcium.

033

PREPARATION
5 minutes

STORAGE
Make on the day. Keep chilled until ready to eat (see page 17).

SERVE THIS WITH...
avocado slices
Chewy Date Bar (see page 127)
grapes

HEALTH BENEFITS
Salmon provides rich amounts of vitamin D, which is good for the skin and valuable for people who get little of this important vitamin from sunlight.

cajun salmon & cucumber roll

Canned salmon sandwiches are reminiscent of days gone by, but a simple sprinkling of spices adds a new twist. Try to buy wild Alaskan salmon from sustainable sources.

60g/2¼oz canned salmon,
    skin removed
¼–½ tsp mixed Cajun spices
squeeze of lemon juice

crusty brown roll
1 tsp mayonnaise
5 slices cucumber

1 Spoon the salmon into a bowl and mix with the spices. Squeeze some lemon juice over the top.
2 Cut the roll in half and spread one side with the mayonnaise. Spoon the salmon on top, followed by the cucumber slices. Place the other half of the roll on top.

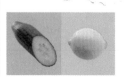

smoked salmon spirals

Simply by experimenting with different shapes and sizes, you can make a sandwich more interesting and fun. The lemon cream cheese adds a new twist to this classic filling.

1 tbsp low-fat cream cheese
squeeze of lemon juice
1 slice wholemeal bread

1 slice white bread
slices of smoked salmon or trout
freshly ground black pepper

1 Mix the cream cheese with the lemon juice and season with pepper.
2 Cut the crusts off both slices of bread and spread the lemon cream cheese over one slice. Arrange a layer of fish on the bread and top with the remaining slice of bread.
3 Press down on the sandwich to flatten it slightly, then roll it up tightly into a cylinder shape. Wrap in cling film until ready to slice. Cut the bread into 1cm/½in slices.

SERVES 1

PREPARATION
10 minutes

STORAGE
Make the day before and keep in the fridge overnight. Slice on the day. Keep chilled until ready to eat (see page 17).

SERVE THIS WITH…
Roasted Red Pepper Hummus (see page 28)
carrot and cucumber sticks
fruit yogurt
raisins

HEALTH BENEFITS
Wholemeal flour provides more fibre, vitamins and minerals than white flour, which loses much of its nutrients during processing – although it is now possible to buy white bread with similar nutrient levels to brown!

Ⓥ

HEALTH BENEFITS
It is recommended that every day we eat a "rainbow" of different-coloured fruit and vegetables. There's good reason for this, because each colour provides a range of nutritious phytochemicals (plant nutrients), vitamins and minerals.

roasted veg & halloumi pitta

Vegetables when roasted seem to lose any trace of bitterness and take on a delicious caramelized sweetness; and they're just as good served cold as hot. Halloumi is a traditional Cypriot cheese that is at its best when griddled or fried quickly in a little oil.

2½ tbsp olive oil
1 tbsp balsamic vinegar
1 small red pepper, seeded
    and cut into 8 slices
1 small courgette,
    sliced lengthways

1 small onion, cut into 8 wedges
2 tomatoes, halved
4 slices halloumi cheese,
    patted dry
2 wholemeal pitta breads

SERVES 2

PREPARATION + COOKING
15 + 35 minutes

STORAGE
Cook the vegetables and
halloumi in advance and keep
in the fridge for up to 3 days.
Assemble on the day.

1 Preheat the oven to 200°C/400°F/Gas 6. Mix together
2 tbsp of the oil and the balsamic vinegar in a shallow dish.
Add the red pepper, courgette, onion and tomatoes and
turn the vegetables to coat them in the oil mixture.
2 Put the vegetables, except the tomatoes, in a roasting
tin. Roast for 20 minutes, turning occasionally, then add
the tomatoes. Return the tin to the oven and cook for
another 10–15 minutes until the vegetables are tender
and slightly blackened around the edges. Leave to cool.
3 Meanwhile, wipe the remaining oil over a griddle or
frying pan and heat until hot. Griddle or fry the halloumi for
a few minutes, turning once, until beginning to turn golden.
4 Slice each pitta lengthways, leaving each end intact, and
open out to make a large pocket. Divide the vegetables and
halloumi between the pittas and close to encase the filling.

SERVE THIS WITH...
Soy-coated Nuts & Seeds
 (see page 20)
Mango Fool (see page 123)
fruit

**The balsamic
vinegar helps to
caramelize the
vegetables and
gives a slight
sweetness.**

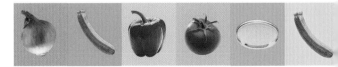

V O

pipérade pitta

Pipérade is a French Basque recipe based on scrambled eggs with pepper and tomatoes.

SERVES 1

PREPARATION + COOKING
10 + 4 minutes

STORAGE
Make on the day.

SERVE THIS WITH…
Carrot, Raisin & Pinenut Salad (see page 77)
fresh berries and natural yogurt
dried apricots

HEALTH BENEFITS
Red pepper has three times the amount of vitamin C and nine times the amount of beta-carotene that its green counterpart contains. It is also sweeter in flavour, which tends to appeal more to children.

1 tbsp olive oil
2.5cm/1in wide strip of
   red pepper, diced
1 tomato, halved, seeded
   and diced
1 spring onion, finely chopped

1 tbsp milk
2 free-range eggs,
   lightly beaten
salt
freshly ground black pepper
wholemeal pitta bread

1 Heat the oil in a frying pan and fry the pepper gently for 1 minute, then add the tomato and spring onion and cook for another minute.
2 Mix the milk into the beaten eggs, season, and add to the pan. Cook until the egg is scrambled (about 2 minutes), stirring constantly with a wooden spoon to stop it sticking.
3 Warm the pitta slightly to make opening it easier. Cut in half crossways then spoon the piperade inside. Leave to cool before wrapping.

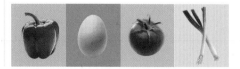

kofta pitta pockets

These lamb kofta are lightly spiced to give them a Moroccan twist.

1 wholemeal pitta
1 tbsp Roasted Aubergine Dip
    (see page 32) or Tzatziki
    (see page 34)
mixed salad leaves
slices of tomato

Kofta:
225g/8oz lean minced lamb

1 shallot, grated
1 clove garlic, crushed
¼ tsp ground cinnamon
1 tsp ground cumin
½ tsp ground coriander
olive oil, for brushing
salt
freshly ground black pepper

1 Put the lamb in a mixing bowl and break it up with a fork. Add the shallot, garlic and spices, season and mix well.
2 Preheat the grill to medium. Shape the lamb mixture into 12 walnut-sized balls. Line a grill rack with foil and lightly brush with oil. Grill the kofta for 8–10 minutes, turning occasionally, until golden. Leave to cool, then refrigerate.
3 Warm the pitta slightly to make it easier to open out. Cut in half crossways to make two pockets, then spread a little of your chosen dip (or you could use mayo, ketchup, relish, mashed avocado or hummus) inside each pocket.
4 Place a few lettuce leaves and slices of tomato in each pocket, followed by two kofta, which can be left whole or cut in half for easier eating.

MAKES 12 KOFTA (4 PER SERVING)

PREPARATION + COOKING
20 + 10 minutes

STORAGE
Make the kofta in advance and keep in the fridge for up to 3 days or freeze for up to 1 month. Assemble on the day. Keep chilled until ready to eat (see page 17).

SERVE THIS WITH...
Melon & Halloumi Salad
 (see page 78)
natural yogurt with honey
fruit

HEALTH BENEFITS
Spices have been prescribed for their digestive properties for hundreds of years. They also have antibacterial qualities.

SERVES 1

PREPARATION
10 minutes

STORAGE
Make the day before and keep in the fridge overnight. Keep chilled until ready to eat (see page 17).

SERVE THIS WITH…
Savoury Spicy Popcorn (see page 21)
cherry tomatoes
Custard Tartlet (see page 135)
fruit

HEALTH BENEFITS
As with other meat products, you get what you pay for, so it really is worth splashing out on good-quality ham, which will have fewer additives.

ham roll-ups

A ham sandwich with a difference: it looks good, is easy to make and takes the humble ham sandwich to a new dimension! You need a square loaf for the roll-ups to work.

2 thin slices square Granary loaf
a little butter
½ tsp mild mustard or chutney of choice
2 slices good-quality cooked

ham, roughly the same size as the bread
2 long, thin sticks cucumber (the same length as each slice of bread), seeded

1 Remove the crusts from each slice of bread, then flatten them slightly by pressing down with your fingers. Mix the butter and mustard or chutney together in a bowl, then spread over the bread.

2 Lay a slice of ham on each slice of bread and place the cucumber diagonally across the ham.

3 Starting from one corner, roll each slice up tightly and place seam-side down on a board. Cut each roll-up in half at an angle, then wrap in cling film to keep their shape.

tuna quesadilla

A great alternative to the usual tuna sarnie, this quesadilla can be made in two different ways: either folded into a parcel or cut into wedges.

2 slices mozzarella cheese
1 small soft flour tortilla
3–4 tbsp canned tuna, drained

2 slices tomato
olive oil, for brushing
freshly ground black pepper

1 Place the mozzarella in the centre of the tortilla. Top with the tuna and tomato and fold in the sides of the tortilla to make a square parcel.

2 Brush a frying pan with olive oil. Place the parcel seam-side down in the pan and fry over a low heat for about 3 minutes, turning once, until golden. Leave to cool before wrapping.

3 Alternatively, sandwich the filling between two tortillas, cook on both sides in a lightly oiled frying pan until the cheese melts and the tortillas are slightly golden and crisp, then cut into wedges.

SERVES 1

PREPARATION + COOKING
5 + 3 minutes

STORAGE
Make on the day. Keep chilled until ready to eat (see page 17).

SERVE THIS WITH...
Pear & Ham Bundles
  (see page 24)
carrot sticks
Winter Fruit Salad (see page 122)

HEALTH BENEFITS
Mozzarella's fresh, mild flavour makes it popular with children, and as an added bonus it's low in fat.

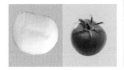

chicken tikka naan

SERVES 1

PREPARATION + COOKING
15 + 4 minutes + marinating

STORAGE
Prepare the chicken in advance and keep in the fridge for up to 3 days or freeze for up to 1 month (unless the chicken was frozen). Assemble on the day. Keep chilled until ready to eat (see page 17).

SERVE THIS WITH...
Soy-coated Nuts & Seeds (see page 20)
cucumber and celery sticks
Cinnamon-spiced Apples (see page 120)

HEALTH BENEFITS
Researchers have found that people who eat garlic on a regular basis are less likely to catch a cold than those who do not.

If you don't have time to make the chicken tikka recipe below, you can buy ready-made chicken tikka from supermarkets.

1 small skinless chicken
    breast, cut into strips
olive oil, for brushing
1 small naan bread
crisp salad leaves

Marinade:
3 tbsp thick natural bio yogurt
1 clove garlic, crushed
1 tbsp tikka curry paste

Yogurt dip:
1 tbsp thick natural bio yogurt
1 tsp chopped fresh mint

1 Mix together the ingredients for the marinade in a shallow dish. Add the chicken strips to the dish and spoon the marinade over until they are coated. Leave to marinate in the fridge for 1 hour, or overnight if preferred.
2 Preheat the grill to medium-high and line a grill pan with foil. Brush the foil with oil and place the marinated chicken on top. Grill for 3–4 minutes on each side until cooked through. Leave to cool then refrigerate.
3 Mix together the yogurt and mint. Split the naan in half, leaving one side attached. Place the chicken in the naan, followed by a few lettuce leaves, then spoon over the yogurt and mint and close up.

roast chicken & avocado focaccia

This is a great way to use up any leftovers from the Sunday roast, so feel free to swap the chicken for any type of roasted meat you have to hand – or indeed a nut roast would work equally well. You could add a few lettuce, watercress or rocket leaves.

½ small avocado,
    stone removed
1 tsp lemon juice
2 tsp mayonnaise
salt

freshly ground black pepper
focaccia, about 10cm/4in
    square (preferably the
    roasted red pepper variety)
few slices roast chicken

1 Scoop the avocado out of its skin into a bowl. Mash with the lemon juice and mayonnaise. Season to taste.
2 Cut the focaccia in half crossways. Spread the avocado over one half of the focaccia. Top with a few slices of chicken, then the other half of the focaccia.

SERVES 1

PREPARATION
10 minutes

STORAGE
Prepare the avocado the day before and keep in the fridge overnight. Assemble on the day.

SERVE THIS WITH…
Apple Coleslaw (see page 76)
Apricot Cookie (see page 136)
fruit

HEALTH BENEFITS
Avocados are almost a complete food, providing small amounts of protein, carbohydrate and beneficial monounsaturated fats. They also contain the highest concentration of vitamin E of any fruit.

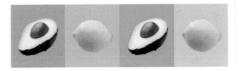

SERVES 1

PREPARATION
5 minutes

STORAGE
Make the falafel in advance and keep in the fridge for up to 3 days or freeze for up to 1 month. Assemble on the day.

SERVE THIS WITH...
Tabbouleh (see page 90)
Apricot & Cashew Nut Bar (see page 128)
fruit

HEALTH BENEFITS
Canned beans are a more convenient alternative to dried pulses, since they don't require lengthy soaking and cooking, but they still contain significant amounts of fibre, which is vital for a healthy digestive system.

falafel & hummus lavash

Lavash is a Middle Eastern flatbread that makes an ideal wrap for all types of fillings. If you can't find one, then a soft flour tortilla will more than do. Or why not serve a falafel like a vegetarian burger in a small seeded bun?

1 lavash
1–2 tbsp Roasted Red Pepper Hummus (see page 28) or Creamy Guacamole (see page 31)

1 Falafel (see page 104)
few sprigs of rocket or watercress

1 Cut the lavash to the size of a small tortilla. Spread the hummus or guacamole over the lavash, then place the falafel in the centre.

2 Arrange the rocket or watercress on top, then fold in the bottom and sides to make a pocket, leaving the top open.

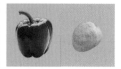

cool dogs

This healthier alternative to the hot dog or sausage roll is best made with good-quality, high-meat-content organic sausages and a soft wholemeal tortilla. The caramelized onions add a delicious sweet moistness but can be replaced with a dollop of good old ketchup, guacamole or hummus, if preferred.

2 good-quality chipolata
   sausages or vegetarian
   alternative
2 tsp olive oil

1 small onion, thinly sliced
1 tsp balsamic vinegar
mild mustard, for spreading
1 soft wholemeal tortilla

1 Preheat the grill to medium-high and line the grill pan with foil. Grill the sausages for about 20 minutes, turning occasionally, until cooked through and golden.
2 Meanwhile, heat the oil in a frying pan and fry the onion over a medium-low heat for about 10 minutes, stirring frequently. Pour in the balsamic vinegar and cook the onions for another 5–8 minutes until golden and glossy.
3 Spread a little mustard over the tortilla, then cut it in half. Divide the onions between the tortilla halves and top each one with a sausage. Fold in the rounded end of each tortilla half and roll up to encase the sausage.

SERVES 1

PREPARATION + COOKING
10 + 20 minutes

STORAGE
Cook in advance and keep in the fridge for up to 3 days. Assemble on the day. Keep chilled until ready to eat (see page 17).

SERVE THIS WITH..
Cheesy Celery Sticks
 (see page 22)
pretzels
Carrot Cake (see page 134)
fruit

HEALTH BENEFITS
Making onions a staple ingredient in your family's diet may greatly reduce the risk of several common cancers.

044

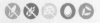

omelette wrap

HEALTH BENEFITS
Eggs provide valuable amounts of iron. A shortage of this mineral is relatively common and has been associated with delays in development and poor concentration.

However much we all like bread, it can become a bit dull if eaten every day. This recipe replaces a flour tortilla with an omelette wrap, which is rolled around crunchy, oriental-flavoured vegetables. The prawns are optional, and you could replace them with toasted sesame seeds, if you prefer.

1 tsp sunflower oil

2 free-range eggs,
   lightly beaten

1 spring onion, cut into long,
   thin strips

¼ red pepper, seeded and cut
   into thin strips

2 sugar snap peas, sliced
   diagonally lengthways

55g/2oz/½ cup small cooked
   prawns (optional)

1cm/½in piece fresh ginger,
   peeled and grated

¼ tsp toasted sesame oil

1 tsp tamari (wheat-free
   soy sauce)

SERVES 1

PREPARATION + COOKING
10 + 3 minutes

STORAGE
Make the omelette the day
before, wrap and keep flat in the
fridge overnight. Assemble on
the day.

SERVE THIS WITH...
rice cakes
Apricot & Cashew Nut Bar
 (see page 128)
fruit

1 Heat the oil in a frying pan. Pour the beaten egg into
the pan and swirl it around so that it covers the bottom.
When the egg begins to set, draw the edges toward the
centre using a wooden spoon, allowing the raw egg to run
into the space. Cook for about 2 minutes until the egg is
set. Slide the omelette on to a plate and leave to cool.

2 Put the spring onion, red pepper, sugar snap peas,
prawns, if using, and ginger in a bowl. Pour the sesame
oil and tamari over them and toss until they are coated.

3 Arrange the vegetables and prawns down the centre of
the omelette, then roll up and cut in half.

Tamari, a by-
product of miso,
is a type of soy
sauce suitable for
gluten-intolerant
people.

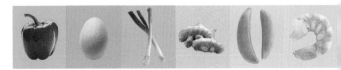

SERVES 1

PREPARATION + COOKING
10 + 2 minutes

STORAGE
Make the stir-fry the day before
and keep in the fridge overnight.
Strain off any liquid and assemble
on the day. Keep chilled until
ready to eat (see page 17).

SERVE THIS WITH...
Chinese Noodle Salad
 (see page 85)
natural yogurt with honey
lychees

HEALTH BENEFITS
Red meat is one of the best
sources of easily absorbed iron.
Make sure you buy good-quality,
lean, organic meat.

oriental beef wrap

A wrap with a difference – a crisp lettuce leaf
rather than a tortilla encases this Chinese beef.

2 tsp sesame oil
1 clove garlic, chopped
few slivers fresh ginger
100g/3½oz lean beef,
 cut into strips
2 tsp tamari (wheat-free
 soy sauce)
1 tbsp orange juice

2 iceberg lettuce leaves
1 spring onion, shredded
5cm/2in piece cucumber,
 seeded and cut into strips
¼ red pepper, seeded and cut
 into strips
coriander leaves (optional)
freshly ground black pepper

1 Heat a wok over a high heat and add the sesame oil,
garlic, ginger and beef, then stir-fry for 1 minute. Add the
tamari and orange juice and stir-fry for another minute
until the liquid has reduced and thickened. Leave to cool.
2 Open out the lettuce leaves and divide the beef between
them, spooning it down one half of each leaf. Top with the
spring onion, cucumber, pepper and coriander, if using.
3 Season and roll each leaf up to make a parcel. Cut each
roll in half diagonally.

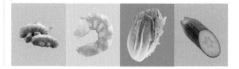

rice paper rolls

These rolls use pork, but you could use any leftover roast meat or the beef stir-fry opposite.

1cm/½in piece fresh ginger, peeled and grated
1 tbsp tamari (wheat-free soy sauce), plus extra for dipping
1 tsp sesame oil
4 spring onions, shredded
1 carrot, cut into matchsticks

½ yellow pepper, seeded and cut into thin strips
20 medium rice paper wrappers
5 tbsp gluten-free hoisin sauce
55g/2oz rice vermicelli noodles, cooked
400g/14oz roast pork, cut into long, thin strips

1 Mix together the ginger, tamari and sesame oil in a bowl. Add the spring onions, carrot and pepper and turn to coat.
2 Fill a heatproof bowl with just-boiled water. Put two rice paper wrappers on top of one another and soak in the water for 20 seconds or until they are pliable and opaque. Carefully remove using a spatula (they are very delicate), drain for a second and place flat on a plate.
3 Spread a teaspoonful of hoisin sauce over a wrapper, then top with a small bundle of noodles, a few strips of pork and a few strips of spring onion, carrot and pepper.
4 Roll the wrapper around the filling, folding in the edges to seal. Repeat using the remaining wrappers and filling ingredients. Serve with a little pot of tamari to dip into.

MAKES 10

PREPARATION + COOKING
20 + 2 minutes

STORAGE
Make in advance and keep in the fridge for up to 3 days or freeze for up to 1 month. Keep chilled until ready to eat (see page 17).

SERVE THIS WITH...
Soy-coated Nuts & Seeds (see page 20)
cookie
fruit

HEALTH BENEFITS
Rice paper wrappers are ideal for those who are allergic to wheat or are gluten-intolerant.

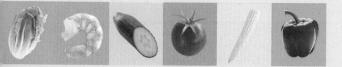

SALADS

The secret of the success of a lunchbox salad is to keep it cool, fresh and crisp. Certain salads, such as those made with pasta, beans, potatoes, grains and noodles, withstand being transported much better than others, being more robust than those containing delicate leaves. The latter are best dressed just before eating, so if possible pack a small pot of dressing that can be poured over when needed. Many of the salads in this chapter are substantial enough to be a main meal, particularly those that contain a carbohydrate element, such as pasta or beans, along with protein such as meat, seafood or cheese. Salads made with grains, meat and seafood need to be kept cool, so store in an insulated lunchbox with ice-pack or in a fridge, if possible.

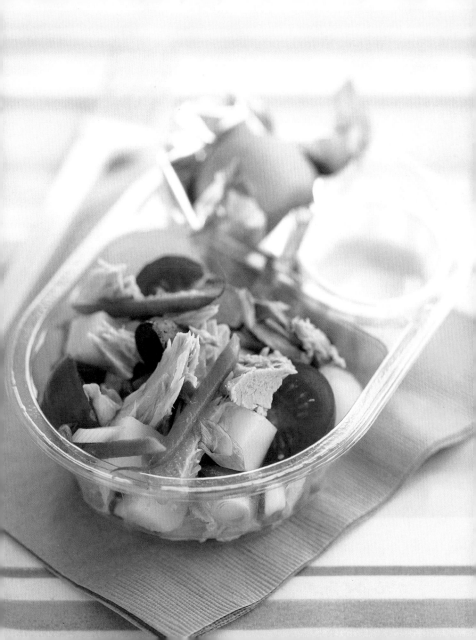

(V) (X) (X) (X) (O)

apple coleslaw

SERVES 4

PREPARATION
10 minutes

STORAGE
Make in advance and keep in the fridge for up to 3 days.

SERVE THIS WITH...
Mini Tart (see page 102)
Apricot & Cashew Nut Bar
 (see page 128)
fruit

HEALTH BENEFITS
Cabbage when served raw is not only more nutritious than cooked, but is generally more acceptable to children, especially when finely shredded and lightly coated in a dressing. Numerous studies highlight cabbage's antiviral and antibacterial properties, and it is also believed to protect the body against certain forms of cancer.

This is nothing like shop-bought coleslaw, in which insipid vegetables come dripping in an additive-laden dressing. Crisp, crunchy and packed with vitamins, this colourful salad will awaken the tastebuds. You could also sprinkle a handful of toasted seeds over the top.

55g/2oz red or white
 cabbage, grated
1 large carrot, grated
2 spring onions, finely sliced
1 apple, cored and grated

Dressing:
1 tbsp extra-virgin olive oil
1 tsp lemon juice
1 tbsp mayonnaise

1 Mix the cabbage, carrot, onions and apple together in a bowl.
2 Whisk the oil and lemon juice together, then stir in the mayonnaise. Spoon the dressing over the salad and stir until combined.

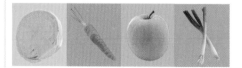

Ⓥ Ⓧ Ⓧ Ⓐ Ⓟ

carrot, raisin & pinenut salad

Pinenuts are not nuts at all but the seeds of the Stone Pine tree, which is native to the Mediterranean region. They have the highest protein content of all seeds, and nuts too.

1 heaped tbsp pinenuts
1 large carrot, grated
1 heaped tbsp raisins

Dressing:
1½ tbsp extra-virgin olive oil
1 tsp fresh lemon juice
¼ tsp ground cumin

1 Put the pinenuts in a dry frying pan and toast them over a medium heat for about 3 minutes, turning them occasionally, until slightly golden – take care as they can easily burn. Leave the nuts to cool, then place in a bowl with the carrot and raisins.
2 Mix together the dressing ingredients and pour over the salad before serving, turning until coated in the dressing.

SERVES 2

PREPARATION + COOKING
10 + 3 minutes

STORAGE
Make in advance and keep in the fridge for up to 3 days.

SERVE THIS WITH...
Chicken Strips with Satay Dip
  (see page 26)
wholemeal bread
Strawberry Crunch Pot
  (see page 124)

HEALTH BENEFITS
Raisins are a good source of potassium, which helps to regulate fluid levels in the body, along with energy-boosting iron.

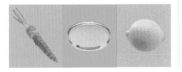

049

(V) (X) (X)

melon & halloumi salad

Melon works particularly well with slightly salty cheeses, such as halloumi, feta or Cheddar, or meats such as crispy bacon, salami or ham.

SERVES 1

PREPARATION + COOKING
5 + 6 minutes

STORAGE
Make the day before and keep in the fridge overnight.

SERVE THIS WITH...
slices of pitta bread
hummus
Date & Pecan Brownie
  (see page 133)
fruit

HEALTH BENEFITS
The vibrant orange colour of the Charentais or Cantaloupe melon comes from lycopene, which can help protect the skin from the sun's UV rays. These melons also contain beneficial amounts of beta-carotene.

olive oil, for brushing
3 slices halloumi cheese,
  rinsed and patted dry
1 large wedge melon
mint leaves, chopped (optional)

Dressing:
1 tbsp extra-virgin olive oil,
  plus extra for brushing
1 tsp fresh lemon juice

1 Lightly brush a frying pan with oil and heat. When the pan is hot, put the halloumi in the pan and cook for about 2–3 minutes on each side until light golden. Cut each slice into quarters.
2 Remove the skin from the melon and cut it into chunks. Combine with the halloumi.
3 Combine the dressing ingredients and pour over the salad with some mint, if using, turning to coat the leaves.

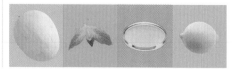

(V) (X) (X)

greek salad

Children like this chunky salad because all the ingredients are easily identifiable. It's also a salad that is easily transportable because it doesn't suffer when it gets swung around!

85g/3oz feta cheese, rinsed,
    patted dry and cut into cubes
2 tomatoes, seeded and
    cut into chunks
10cm/4in piece cucumber,
    cut into chunks
¼ small red onion, thinly sliced

8 black olives (optional)
1 tbsp chopped mint or oregano
    leaves (optional)

Dressing:
2 tbsp extra-virgin olive oil
2 tsp fresh lemon juice

1 Put the feta in a bowl with the tomatoes, cucumber, red onion and olives, if using.
2 Whisk together the oil and lemon juice and pour the dressing over the salad. Turn to coat the salad in the dressing and sprinkle with the mint or oregano, if using.

SERVES 2

PREPARATION
10 minutes

STORAGE
Make in advance and keep in the fridge for up to 2 days.

SERVE THIS WITH...
Roasted Aubergine Dip
 (see page 32)
toasted wedges of tortilla
Chewy Date Bar (see page 127)
fruit

HEALTH BENEFITS
A popular vegetable with the Greeks and Romans, cucumber is a good source of potassium and may help to relieve high blood pressure.

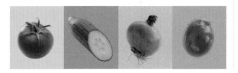

051

Ⓥ Ⓧ Ⓧ

italian flag salad

Tricolore is a classic Italian salad that uses, patriotically, the same colours as its national flag. This version is able to withstand being carried about, but pack the avocado tightly in a container so that it is unable to slip around.

SERVES 1

PREPARATION
10 minutes

STORAGE
Prepare the tomato and mozzarella the day before and keep in the fridge overnight. Assemble on the day.

SERVE THIS WITH...
Simple Mini Pizza (see page 100)
muffin
fruit

HEALTH BENEFITS
Avocados provide more than 25 essential nutrients, including vitamin E, B vitamins, folic acid, lutein and fibre.

½ avocado, stone removed
lemon juice, for brushing
1 tomato, seeded and diced
40g/1½oz mozzarella cheese,
    cut into chunks
basil leaves (optional)

Dressing:
1 tbsp extra-virgin olive oil
1 tsp balsamic vinegar
freshly ground black pepper

1 Place the avocado in a plastic container that has a lid, making sure it is quite a tight fit, then brush a little lemon juice over the top to prevent it turning brown.
2 Arrange the tomato and mozzarella on top of the avocado, then sprinkle with a few basil leaves, if using.
3 Whisk together the dressing ingedients, store in a little lidded pot and pour over the salad just before serving.

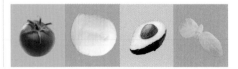

super salad

The word "super" is justly earned by this salad: sprouted beans and seeds are a nutritional powerhouse providing surprisingly high amounts of protein as well as vitamins and minerals. Bags of mixed sprouted beans are perfect for this: look for fresh, crisp sprouts.

85g/3oz mixed sprouted beans and seeds, such as alfalfa, chickpeas, mung beans, aduki beans and lentils
4 radishes, thinly sliced
1 carrot, grated
½ small red onion, diced

Dressing:
1 tbsp extra-virgin olive oil
2 tsp sesame oil
1 tsp grated fresh ginger
1 tsp tamari (wheat-free soy sauce)
2 tsp rice vinegar or lemon juice

1 Mix together the ingredients for the dressing; set aside.
2 Put the sprouted beans and seeds, radishes, carrot and red onion in a bowl. Pour the dressing over the salad and turn to coat the ingredients in the dressing.

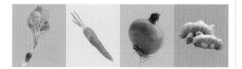

SERVES 2

PREPARATION
10 minutes

STORAGE
Make the day before and keep in the fridge overnight, with the dressing separate. Assemble on the day.

SERVE THIS WITH...
Tuna & Onion Tortilla
(see page 111)
Custard Tartlet (see page 135)
fruit

HEALTH BENEFITS
Unlike most fruits and vegetables, whose nutrient levels start to diminish as soon as they are picked, the concentration of vitamins and minerals in sprouted beans and seeds continues to increase when sprouted. There are around 30 per cent more B vitamins and 60 per cent more vitamin C in the sprout than in the bean or seed in its original state.

mixed bean salad

HEALTH BENEFITS
Foods rich in vitamin C, such as the apple and red pepper in this salad, will help your child's body to absorb the iron found in the pulses.

This salad is incredibly versatile: treat the beans as a base and add any favourite fruit, vegetables, nuts, seeds or herbs you have to hand or that you know will go down well – the more colourful the better.

400g/14oz/scant 3-cup can
    mixed beans, drained
    and rinsed
1 red pepper, seeded
    and diced
1 stick celery, sliced
2 spring onions, sliced
2 tbsp chopped mint (optional)
1 apple, cored and diced
squeeze of lemon juice

Dressing:
2 tbsp extra-virgin olive oil
2 tsp white wine vinegar
½ tsp mustard powder
¼ tsp sugar
salt
freshly ground black pepper

SERVES 4

PREPARATION
10 minutes

STORAGE
Make in advance and keep in the
fridge for up to 2 days.

SERVE THIS WITH...
Tandoori Chicken Drumstick
  (see page 117) or
  hard-boiled egg
mini pitta bread
dried fruit

1 Mix together the dressing ingredients in a small bowl.
2 Put the beans in a serving bowl with the red pepper,
celery, spring onions and mint, if using.
3 Put the diced apple in another bowl, add the lemon juice,
toss to prevent the apple browning, then add to the salad.
4 Pour the dressing over the salad, then toss until
everything is mixed together.

**Aromatic mint
adds a fresh,
sweet flavour
to this salad
and also aids
digestion.**

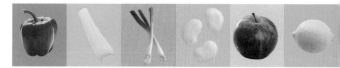

ham, bean & pineapple salad

This chunky, robust salad has a good mix of sweet and savoury flavours. The fruit adds a delicious sweetness, which always goes down well with children, as well as a nutritional boost. Choose pineapple canned in natural juice rather than syrup.

SERVES 2

PREPARATION
10 minutes

STORAGE
Make in advance and keep in the fridge for up to 3 days. Keep chilled until ready to eat (see page 17).

SERVE THIS WITH...
pitta bread
Summer Pudding (see page 130)
fruit

HEALTH BENEFITS
Beans count in the "five-a-day" guidelines and also provide plenty of slow-release energy.

175g/6oz canned pineapple, cut into chunks
150g/5½oz thickly cut good-quality ham, cubed
100g/3½oz canned cannellini beans, drained and rinsed

Dressing:
1 tbsp natural juice from the pineapple
1½ tbsp extra-virgin olive oil
2 tsp white wine vinegar
½ tsp Dijon mustard

1 Mix together the ingredients for the dressing.
2 Put the pineapple, ham and beans in a bowl, then pour the dressing over the top. Toss the salad well to coat it thoroughly in the dressing.

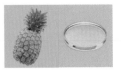

V ☺ ⊙ ☯

chinese noodle salad

Noodles are fun to eat and are just as good cold as hot. The oriental-style dressing not only has a delicious ginger and sesame flavour, but also prevents the noodles sticking together, which they can do when cold. For this reason it's best to pour the dressing over while they are warm.

70g/2½oz/heaped ½ cup
    medium egg noodles
1 carrot, cut into thin strips
5cm/2in piece cucumber,
    seeded and cut
    into matchsticks
2 tomatoes, seeded and diced
2 spring onions, finely sliced
3 tbsp chopped coriander or
    basil (optional)
1 tbsp toasted sesame seeds

Dressing:
1 tbsp olive oil
1 tsp toasted sesame oil
1 tsp soy sauce
1 tsp grated fresh ginger
1 small clove garlic, crushed
1 tsp lemon juice

SERVES 2

PREPARATION + COOKING
15 + 5 minutes

STORAGE
Make in advance and keep in the fridge for up to 3 days.

SERVE THIS WITH...
Tofu Bites (see page 105)
fresh berries and natural yogurt

HEALTH BENEFITS
Noodles are low in fat. They are also an excellent source of selenium, thiamine and folate, and a good source of niacin. Niacin and thiamine are both B vitamins; they work in tandem and are essential for the production of energy.

1 Cook the noodles following the packet instructions; drain and refresh under cold running water. Meanwhile, mix together the ingredients for the dressing. Pour it over the noodles and leave to cool.
2 Put the noodles, carrot, cucumber, tomatoes, spring onions and coriander or basil, if using, in a bowl, then toss with your hands to mix. Sprinkle with the sesame seeds.

Ⓥ Ⓞ ⓓ

pesto pasta salad

Popular with kids, pesto makes a quick and easy dressing when mixed with mayonnaise. The small florets of broccoli add lots of goodness, but may not appeal to all children, so you can swap them for sweetcorn or diced pepper instead. New potatoes can replace the pasta.

SERVES 2

PREPARATION + COOKING
10 + 12 minutes

STORAGE
Make the day before and keep in the fridge overnight.

SERVE THIS WITH...
Pear & Ham Bundles
 (see page 24)
cookie
fruit

HEALTH BENEFITS
Surprisingly, frozen peas are often more nutritious than fresh. This is because freezing takes place soon after picking, before the vitamin values have fallen. Peas provide significant amounts of protein, vitamins B and C and iron, making them a good choice for vegetarians.

100g/3½oz/1 cup farfalle pasta
6 small florets broccoli
55g/2oz frozen petits pois
55g/2oz mature Cheddar cheese,
   cut into small chunks
salt

Dressing:
1 tbsp mayonnaise
1–2 tbsp pesto
squeeze of lemon juice
freshly ground black pepper

1 Bring a large saucepan of salted water to the boil. Add the pasta, stir and cook following the packet instructions until al dente. Drain well and refresh under cold water.
2 Meanwhile, steam the broccoli for 4 minutes until only just tender – it should still be slightly crunchy. Add the peas about 1½ minutes before the end of the cooking time. Refresh the vegetables under cold running water.
3 Mix the dressing ingredients together, adding pesto to taste, and season with pepper. Put the pasta, vegetables and Cheddar in a bowl and spoon the dressing over the top. Turn the salad with a spoon to coat it in the dressing.

prawn pasta salad

A complete meal in a pot, this salad combines protein from the prawns and carbohydrate from the pasta with lots of vitamins and minerals.

100g/3½oz/1 cup pasta shells
115g/4oz cooked peeled small
    prawns, defrosted if frozen
6 cherry tomatoes, quartered
crisp lettuce leaves, such as
    Cos, shredded

Dressing:
1 tbsp mayonnaise
1 tsp lemon juice
1 tbsp tomato ketchup
2 drops Tabasco (optional)
salt
freshly ground black pepper

1 Bring a large saucepan of salted water to the boil. Add the pasta, stir and cook following the packet instructions until al dente. Drain well and refresh under cold water.
2 Put the prawns and tomatoes in a bowl with the pasta and season with pepper.
3 Mix the dressing ingredients together and spoon over the salad. Turn the salad with a spoon to coat it well.
4 Serve the prawn salad on a bed of shredded lettuce.

SERVES 2

PREPARATION + COOKING
10 + 12 minutes

STORAGE
Make in advance and keep in the fridge for up to 2 days. Assemble on the day. Keep chilled until ready to eat (see page 17).

SERVE THIS WITH...
Apricot & Cashew Nut Bar
  (see page 128)
fruit

HEALTH BENEFITS
Prawns are rich in the antioxidant minerals selenium and zinc, which are good for the skin.

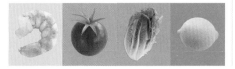

prawn salad lunchbowl

SERVES 1

PREPARATION
10 minutes

STORAGE
Make the day before and keep in the fridge overnight. Assemble on the day. Keep chilled until ready to eat (see page 17).

SERVE THIS WITH…
crusty wholemeal bread
Apple Flapjack (see page 126)
fruit

HEALTH BENEFITS
Canned sweetcorn is a good source of readily usable fibre, as are beans; these help to keep the digestive system working efficiently.

This salad is arranged in distinct, colourful layers, which add to its appeal and flexibility. To keep the layers intact during the school day, pack the salad fairly tightly in an airtight pot.

40g/1½oz crisp lettuce leaves
  such as Cos, thickly sliced
55g/2oz canned beans of
  choice, drained and rinsed
1 carrot, finely grated
6 slices cucumber
3 tbsp canned no-salt, no-sugar
  sweetcorn, drained
115g/4oz cooked peeled prawns

Dressing:
1 tbsp extra-virgin olive oil
2 tsp mayonnaise
½ clove garlic, crushed
1 tsp lemon juice
salt
freshly ground black pepper

1 Mix together the ingredients for the dressing and keep in a small pot until ready to use.
2 Arrange the salad ingredients in layers: salad leaves, beans, carrot, cucumber, sweetcorn and prawns. Spoon the dressing over the salad when ready to eat.

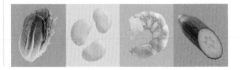

tuna niçoise

Keep the dressing separate and pour it over just before eating; store the remainder in the fridge.

1 large Cos lettuce leaf, roughly sliced
55g/2oz cooked fine green beans, halved
3 cooked small new potatoes, cut into cubes
3 cherry tomatoes, halved
1 spring onion, sliced
6 pitted black olives, halved

150g/5½oz can tuna, drained
1 hard-boiled free-range egg, shell left on

Dressing:
2 tbsp extra-virgin olive oil
1 tsp white wine vinegar
½ clove garlic, crushed
3 tbsp mayonnaise

1 Arrange the Cos lettuce in the bottom of a pot. Place the green beans on top, then add the potatoes.

2 Next, put the tomatoes, spring onion and olives in the pot. Flake the tuna and place it on top. Leave the egg in its shell and wrap in foil.

3 Whisk together the ingredients for the dressing. Put one serving in a small pot or drizzle it over the salad.

4 When ready to eat, peel the egg and serve with the salad.

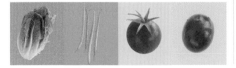

SERVES 1 (DRESSING FOR 4)

PREPARATION
15 minutes

STORAGE
Prepare the ingredients the day before and keep in the fridge overnight. Assemble on the day. Keep chilled until ready to eat (see page 17).

SERVE THIS WITH...
Seeded Dough Balls
  (see page 139)
Mango Fool (see page 123)
fruit

HEALTH BENEFITS
Although canned tuna is not as rich in the beneficial omega-3 fatty acids as fresh tuna, it still provides useful amounts as well as B vitamins (vital for a healthy nervous system and energy metabolism) and selenium.

V

tabbouleh

This is a perfect salad for a lunchbox because it can withstand being carried around and tastes at its best when not over-chilled. Bulghur wheat is most commonly used in this Middle Eastern salad, but you could also try brown rice, couscous and protein-rich quinoa

SERVES 2

PREPARATION + COOKING
10 + 15 minutes

STORAGE
Make in advance and keep in the fridge for up to 3 days. Keep chilled until ready to eat (see page 17).

SERVE THIS WITH...
Falafel & Hummus Lavash
 (see page 68)
Apricot Cookie (see page 136)
fruit

HEALTH BENEFITS
Bulghur wheat has a light, nutty taste and is a better source of nutrients than white flour, as it contains more fibre and selenium.

55g/2oz/⅓ cup bulghur wheat
3 small tomatoes, seeded
 and chopped
2 spring onions, finely chopped
5cm/2in piece cucumber, diced
3 tbsp chopped mint
3 tbsp chopped parsley

salt
freshly ground black pepper

Dressing:
1 tbsp extra-virgin olive oil
2 tbsp lemon juice

1 Put the bulghur wheat in a saucepan and cover it with cold water. Bring to the boil then reduce the heat, cover and simmer for 10–15 minutes until tender. Drain, if necessary, and leave to cool.

2 Put the bulghur wheat in a bowl with the tomatoes, spring onions, cucumber and herbs.

3 Mix together the olive oil and lemon juice and pour the dressing over the salad. Season to taste and turn the salad to coat it in the dressing.

Ⓥ Ⓧ Ⓧ ⊜ ⊜

oriental rice salad

Vary this salad by adding different vegetables, meat or fish to the rice and dressing base.

100g/3½oz/½ cup brown
   basmati rice
½ red pepper, seeded
   and diced
2 spring onions, thinly sliced
3 baby sweetcorn, quartered
2 tbsp toasted sunflower and
   sesame seeds

Dressing:
2 tbsp sunflower oil
1 tbsp fresh apple juice
2 tsp tamari (wheat-free
   soy sauce)
2 tsp rice wine vinegar or
   white wine vinegar
½ tsp Chinese five spice powder
1 tsp clear honey
½–1 tsp grated fresh ginger

1 Put the rice in a pan with plenty of salted water, bring to the boil, then simmer for 10 minutes, or until cooked. Drain, then rinse under cold running water until cold.
2 Put the cooked rice, red pepper, spring onions, baby sweetcorn and toasted seeds in a bowl.
3 Mix together the ingredients for the dressing, then pour over the salad, turning it gently until it is well coated.

SERVES 2

PREPARATION + COOKING
10 + 10 minutes

STORAGE
Make in advance and keep in the fridge for up to 2 days. Keep chilled until ready to eat (see page 17).

SERVE THIS WITH...
Spring Roll (see page 113)
Winter Fruit Salad (see page 122)

HEALTH BENEFITS
Brown rice produces a gentler rise in blood-sugar levels than white rice, potatoes or bread, therefore keeping energy levels steady. Brown rice also has more nutrients than white and is higher in fibre and vitamin B1.

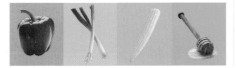

spicy bulghur salad with nectarines

HEALTH BENEFITS
Made from wheat berries, this light, nutty grain is a good source of dietary fibre and B vitamins as well as the immunity-boosting minerals iron and selenium.

Bulghur wheat is easy for children to eat and its mild flavour works well with this lightly spiced dressing. Add halloumi, mozzarella or chicken to introduce some protein to the meal.

100g/3½oz/½ cup
  bulghur wheat
475ml/16fl oz/2 cups
  vegetable stock
1 tbsp olive oil
2 cloves garlic, chopped
1 tsp ground cumin
1 tsp ground coriander

½ tsp ground cinnamon
1 ripe nectarine, halved, stone
  removed and sliced
3 tbsp toasted pinenuts
  (optional)
2 tbsp chopped coriander
  (optional)
freshly ground black pepper

1 Put the bulghur wheat in a saucepan with the stock.
Bring to the boil then reduce the heat, cover and simmer
for 10–15 minutes until the stock is absorbed. Remove
from the heat and leave the pan to stand for 5 minutes
with the lid on.

2 Meanwhile, heat the oil in a frying pan and fry the garlic
for 1 minute, then add the spices and cook for another
minute. Remove from the heat, add the wheat and stir to
coat it in the spices. Transfer to a bowl and leave to cool.

3 Stir in the nectarine, pinenuts and coriander, if using,
and season with pepper.

SERVES 4

PREPARATION + COOKING
10 + 18 minutes

STORAGE
Make in advance and keep in
the fridge for up to 3 days.
Keep chilled until ready to eat
(see page 17).

SERVE THIS WITH...
Cheesy Celery Sticks
 (see page 22)
natural yogurt with honey
fruit

Fresh fruit in
salads adds
a valuable
nutritional boost
and a delicious
sweetness.

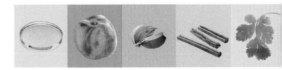

sausage & barley salad

This wholesome, robust salad is easy for children to eat. It's best to use organic sausages with a high meat content to avoid unnecessary additives and fillers.

SERVES 4

PREPARATION + COOKING
soaking + 15 + 20 minutes

STORAGE
Make in advance and keep in the fridge for up to 3 days or freeze for up to 1 month. Keep chilled until ready to eat (see page 17).

SERVE THIS WITH...
celery and carrot sticks
Banana & Blueberry Muffin
  (see page 132)
fruit

HEALTH BENEFITS
Barley has a mild, sweet flavour and chewy texture; its fibre content has been shown to help prevent constipation as well as heart disease and bowel disorders, including colon and rectal cancer.

100g/3½oz/heaped ½ cup
  pearl barley
6 good-quality sausages, or
  vegetarian alternative
2 tbsp olive oil

2 cloves garlic, finely chopped
1 tsp dried oregano
4 tbsp canned tomatoes
salt
freshly ground black pepper

1 Soak the barley for 6 hours or overnight; drain and rinse.
2 Preheat the grill to medium and line the grill pan with foil. Grill the sausages, turning them occasionally, for 20 minutes until cooked through and browned. Leave to cool.
3 Meanwhile, heat the oil in a frying pan and fry the garlic for 1 minute, stirring. Add the oregano, tomatoes and barley and cook for 10 minutes, stirring occasionally. Remove from the heat and leave to cool.
4 Slice the sausages and stir into the barley mixture.

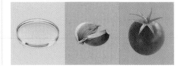

Ⓥ Ⓧ Ⓧ

spicy sweet potatoes

These are a good introduction to curry flavours for children who may be reluctant to try spicy foods. The dressing is also delicious with prawns or chunks of poached chicken, or with a hard-boiled egg.

280g/10oz orange-fleshed
    sweet potato, peeled and cut
    into bite-sized chunks
1 stick celery, thinly sliced

Dressing:
1 tbsp low-fat natural
    bio yogurt
¾ tsp tandoori spice mix or
    curry powder
1 tsp smooth mango chutney
squeeze of lemon juice

1 Cook the sweet potato in plenty of boiling water for about 8–10 minutes until tender. Drain and refresh the potato under cold running water to stop it cooking any further.
2 Meanwhile, mix the dressing ingredients in a bowl.
3 Put the potato and celery in a bowl, spoon the dressing over the top and turn the salad with a spoon to coat it well.

SERVES 2

PREPARATION + COOKING
10 + 10 minutes

STORAGE
Make in advance and keep in the fridge for up to 3 days.

SERVE THIS WITH...
Tandoori Chicken Drumstick
  (see page 117)
cucumber sticks
Chewy Date Bar (see page 127)
fruit

HEALTH BENEFITS
Containing far more vitamins than ordinary potatoes, sweet potatoes are a good source of iron, beta-carotene and vitamin C and are the only low-fat food with a significant vitamin-E content.

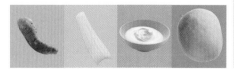

SERVES 2

PREPARATION + COOKING
15 + 12 minutes

STORAGE
Make the day before and keep in the fridge overnight. Assemble on the day. Keep chilled until ready to eat (see page 17).

SERVE THIS WITH...
Cheese Scones (see page 138)
cookie
fruit

HEALTH BENEFITS
Mackerel contains significant amounts of omega-3 fatty acids, which are vital for children's developing brains, eyes, skin and nervous system.

smoked mackerel, apple & potato salad

Mackerel is a much underrated oily fish, being healthy, cheap and versatile. When smoked, it makes a protein-rich addition to a salad that works best with a slightly creamy dressing.

250g/9oz new potatoes, scrubbed and halved if large
85g/3oz smoked mackerel fillets (or salmon or trout)
1 small red apple, cored and diced
2 sticks celery, finely chopped

Dressing:
1½ tbsp mayonnaise
1 tbsp extra-virgin olive oil
2 tsp creamed horseradish
1 tsp lemon juice, plus a little extra for the apple

1 Cook the potatoes in a pan of boiling water for about 12 minutes, until tender; drain and set aside to cool.
2 Meanwhile, mix together the ingredients for the dressing with 1 tbsp water until smooth and creamy.
3 Peel the skin off the mackerel and break into large chunks. Toss the apple in a little lemon juice to prevent it turning brown. Put the apple in a bowl with the mackerel, potatoes and celery.
4 Spoon the dressing over the top. Turn the salad until it is coated in the dressing.

chicken caesar salad

This is a Caesar salad with a difference: the dressing has been adapted to make it more child-friendly and it also contains new potatoes, making it a nutritionally balanced lunch.

250g/9oz new potatoes, scrubbed, and halved if large
2 tsp olive oil
150g/5½oz skinless chicken breast, cut into large bite-sized pieces
2 Cos lettuce leaves, shredded
2 tomatoes, seeded and diced

Dressing:
1½ tbsp mayonnaise
1½ tbsp extra-virgin olive oil
2 tsp lemon juice
1 small clove garlic, crushed
½ tsp Dijon mustard
¼ tsp gluten-free Worcestershire sauce
2 tbsp finely grated Parmesan cheeese

1 Cook the potatoes in plenty of boiling water for about 12 minutes, until tender; drain and set aside to cool.
2 Meanwhile, heat the olive oil in a frying pan and fry the chicken for 5–6 minutes, turning occasionally, until golden and cooked through. Leave to cool.
3 Put the dressing ingredients in a blender and process until smooth and creamy.
4 Put the Cos lettuce in a bowl and add the potatoes, tomatoes and chicken. Spoon over enough of the dressing to coat the salad.

SERVES 2

PREPARATION + COOKING
15 + 12 minutes

STORAGE
Make the day before and keep in the fridge overnight. Assemble on the day. Keep chilled until ready to eat (see page 17). The remaining dressing will keep in the fridge for up to 1 week.

SERVE THIS WITH...
a handful of walnuts or pretzels
Carrot Cake (see page 134)
fruit

HEALTH BENEFITS
Potatoes are a popular starchy carbohydrate and contain a higher concentration of vitamins and minerals if the skin is left on.

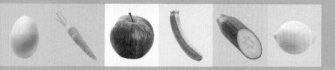

SAVOURIES

Tired of sandwiches? Then this diverse selection of recipes should encourage you to ring the changes. Inspired by some of the cuisines of the world, there's a wide variety to choose from, including Italian Calzone and Simple Mini Pizzas, Spanish Tuna & Onion Tortilla, Chinese Spring Rolls, Japanese Sushi Cones, Middle Eastern Falafel and Indian Tandoori Chicken Drumsticks. Most of the recipes take a little more preparation than a sandwich, but all keep well and can be made in advance, then chilled or frozen for convenience. Importantly, the savouries have been chosen to withstand being transported in a lunchbox and simply need the addition of a salad and vegetable sticks to make them into a complete meal to sustain your child until tea time.

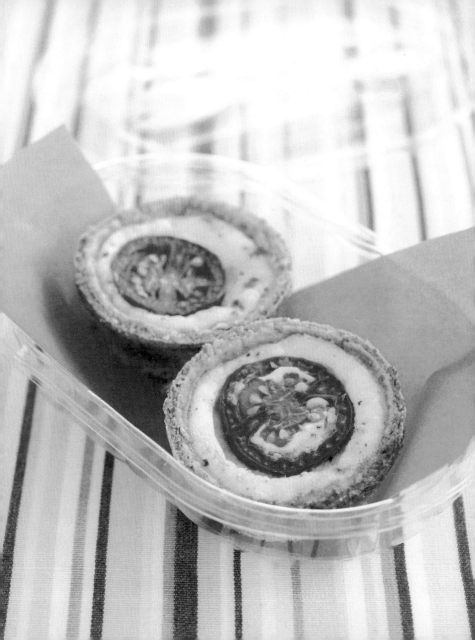

MAKES 6

PREPARATION + COOKING
20 + 25 minutes

STORAGE
Make the day before and keep in the fridge overnight. The dough and sauce can be frozen separately for up to 1 month.

SERVE THIS WITH...
carrot and red pepper sticks
Mango Fool (see page 123)
fruit

HEALTH BENEFITS
Cheese provides valuable amounts of protein and calcium, essential for growing bones and teeth. However, Cheddar is high in saturated fat so try to eat in moderate amounts and choose a mature cheese rather than a mild one, as its strong flavour means that you can use less.

(V)

simple mini pizzas

The dough for these pizzas is made without yeast, which greatly speeds up preparation time.

1 tbsp olive oil
150ml/5fl oz/²/₃ cup passata (sieved tomatoes)
2 tsp tomato purée
½ tsp dried oregano
150g/5½oz ball mozzarella cheese, drained and sliced
50g/2oz mature Cheddar cheese, grated

Dough:
175g/6oz/1½ cups white self-raising flour, plus extra for dusting
100g/3½oz/¾ cup wholemeal self-raising flour
½ tsp salt
150ml/5fl oz/²/₃ cup half-fat milk
4 tbsp olive oil

1 Preheat the oven to 200°C/400°F/Gas 6. Heat the oil in a saucepan and add the passata, tomato purée and oregano, stir and bring to the boil. Half-cover and simmer for 10 minutes, stirring occasionally, until reduced.

2 Sift the flours and salt into a mixing bowl, adding any bran left in the sieve. Make a well in the centre and pour in the milk and oil. Mix with a fork until the ingredients start to come together into a dough (adding a little more milk if dry). Tip the dough out on to a floured work surface and knead briefly until it forms a smooth ball.

3 Divide into six pieces, roll into balls, then flatten into rounds. Place on floured baking sheets. Divide the tomato sauce and cheeses between them. Bake for 10 minutes.

068

(V)

calzone

This portable pizza has its filling safely inside.

1 tbsp olive oil
1 onion, chopped
2 cloves garlic, chopped
1 large carrot, diced
1 small red pepper, seeded
    and diced
250g/9oz vegetarian mince
375ml/13fl oz/1½ cups passata
    (sieved tomatoes)
1 tsp dried oregano
2 tbsp tomato ketchup
freshly ground black pepper

115g/4oz mozzarella cheese,
    cut into small pieces

Dough:
350g/12oz/3 cups white
    self-raising flour, plus extra
    for dusting
200g/7oz/1²/₃ cups wholemeal
    self-raising flour
1 tsp salt
300ml/10fl oz/1¼ cups
    half-fat milk
8 tbsp olive oil

1 Preheat the oven to 200°C/400°F/Gas 6. Heat the oil in a saucepan and fry the onion for 8 minutes, then add the other vegetables and cook for another 3 minutes. Stir in the remaining ingredients and bring to the boil. Simmer for 15 minutes, until reduced. Season well and leave to cool.
2 Make the dough (see Simple Mini Pizzas, opposite), then divide into eight. Roll into thin discs about 12cm/4½in in diameter and divide the sauce and cheese between them.
3 Fold the discs in half, press the edges together and crimp to seal. Prick the top with a fork. Place on floured baking sheets and bake for 10–12 minutes until golden.

MAKES 8

PREPARATION + COOKING
30 + 40 minutes

STORAGE
Make the day before and keep in the fridge overnight.

SERVE THIS WITH…
Italian Flag Salad (see page 80)
grapes

HEALTH BENEFITS
Olive oil contains a higher concentration of monounsaturated fat than any other oil and has a protective role in preventing heart disease.

V O

mini tarts

Small tarts survive better in a lunchbox than individual slices, which are prone to breaking up.

MAKES 8

PREPARATION + COOKING
25 + 22 minutes + chilling

STORAGE
Make in advance and keep in the fridge for up to 1 week or freeze for up to 1 month.

SERVE THIS WITH...
carrot and cucumber sticks
Super Salad (see page 81)
Winter Fruit Salad (see page 122)

HEALTH BENEFITS
Both nutritious and convenient, eggs are now available that are fortified with omega-3 fatty acids, which benefit the nervous system, skin, brain and eyes.

150ml/5fl oz/²/₃ cup milk
4 free-range eggs, lightly beaten
70g/2½oz mature Cheddar
    cheese, grated
1 tomato, sliced into 8 rounds
salt
freshly ground black pepper

Pastry:
200g/7oz/1²/₃ cups wholemeal
    plain flour
100g/3½oz cold unsalted
    butter, cut into small pieces
pinch of salt

1 Sift the flour into a mixing bowl, adding any bran left in the sieve. Rub the butter into the flour using your fingertips until it forms fine breadcrumbs. Pour in 2 tbsp iced water and stir with a fork, then your hands, until it forms a ball. Wrap the pastry in cling film and chill for 30 minutes.

2 Grease an eight-hole deep muffin tin. Roll out the pastry on a floured surface and use to line the holes, leaving the pastry slightly proud at the top. Preheat the oven to 200°C/400°F/Gas 6. Chill the pastry cases for 15 minutes.

3 Bake the pastry cases for 6 minutes, then remove from the oven. Whisk the milk and eggs together and season. Sprinkle the cheese into the cases, add the egg mixture and a slice of tomato and bake for 15 minutes until set.

4 Cool slightly before removing with a palette knife.

ham & egg pies

These simple pies use ham as a base instead of pastry, keeping fat levels down and making them very quick and easy to make. Use a good-quality ham with high-meat, low-water content.

olive oil, for brushing
4 thin slices good-quality ham
4 free-range eggs

1 Preheat the oven to 190°C/375°F/Gas 5. Lightly brush four holes of a deep muffin tin with oil.
2 Arrange a slice of ham in each hole, overlapping the sides where necessary. Carefully trim the top of the ham slices to make them even but leaving the ham slightly above the edge of the tin.
3 Crack an egg into a bowl, then drop it into a ham-lined hollow; repeat with the remaining eggs. Bake for 10–12 minutes until the eggs are set.
4 Leave to cool slightly then lift out the "pies" with a palette knife. Leave to cool completely.

MAKES 4

PREPARATION + COOKING
15 + 12 minutes

STORAGE
Make in advance and keep in the fridge for up to 3 days. Keep chilled until ready to eat (see page 17).

SERVE THIS WITH…
Tabbouleh (see page 90)
Carrot Cake (see page 134)
fruit

HEALTH BENEFITS
Eggs are rich in brain-boosting choline. The body uses choline to produce the neurotransmitter acetylcholine, which has been shown to aid memory.

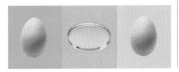

071

⊙⊛⊙⊚

falafel

MAKES 12

PREPARATION + COOKING
15 + 20 minutes + chilling

STORAGE
Make in advance and keep in the fridge for up to 5 days or freeze for up to 1 month.

SERVE THIS WITH...
Falafel & Hummus Lavash (see page 68) or Spicy Bulghur Salad with Nectarines (see page 92)
Apricot Cookie (see page 136)
fruit

HEALTH BENEFITS
A combination of protein provided by the chickpeas and carbohydrate from the flatbread have shown in tests to help students perform better in exams and to help memory recall.

This is a great way to encourage your child to eat beans – other than the baked variety, that is! Serve the falafel wrapped in a flat bread (see page 68) or on their own with a hummus dip.

400g/14oz/scant 3-cup can no-salt, no-sugar chickpeas, drained and rinsed
3 spring onions, finely chopped
2 cloves garlic, crushed
1 tsp ground cumin
1 tsp ground coriander

1–2 tbsp chopped mint (optional)
1 small free-range egg, lightly beaten
salt
freshly ground black pepper
plain flour, for dusting
sunflower oil, for frying

1 Put the chickpeas, spring onions, garlic, cumin, coriander and mint, if using, in a food processor and pulse until the chickpeas are roughly chopped. Add the egg and seasoning and blend until the mixture forms a coarse paste. Chill for 1 hour to allow the mixture to firm up.
2 Form the mixture into 12 walnut-sized balls using floured hands, then lightly dust each ball in flour.
3 Heat 1 tbsp oil in a non-stick frying pan and cook the falafel four at a time (adding more oil when necessary) for 6 minutes, turning them occasionally, until golden all over. Drain on kitchen paper.

V

tofu bites

Cubes of marinated and roasted golden tofu make great nibbles, an addition to a salad such as the Chinese Noodle Salad (see page 85) or a filling for wraps and pitta breads.

4 tbsp black bean sauce
1 tbsp clear honey
1 tbsp soy sauce
2 tsp sesame oil

225g/8oz firm tofu, patted dry
    and cut into 2cm/¾in cubes
sunflower oil, for brushing

1 Mix together the black bean sauce, honey, soy sauce and sesame oil in a shallow dish. Add the tofu and spoon the marinade over until the tofu is completely covered. Leave to marinate for 1 hour, turning the tofu occasionally.
2 Preheat the oven to 180°C/350°F/Gas 4. Lightly brush a roasting tin with oil. Arrange the tofu in the tin and roast for 20 minutes, turning halfway, until golden and slightly crisp all over.

SERVES 4

PREPARATION + COOKING
10 + 20 minutes + marinating

STORAGE
Make in advance and keep in the fridge for up to 3 days.

SERVE THIS WITH...
Chinese Noodle Salad
 (see page 85)
Summer Pudding (see page 130)
fruit

HEALTH BENEFITS
Tofu is made from the soya bean, which is super-nutritious and known as the "meat of the earth" in China, as it is among only a few plant foods that are complete proteins.

*chicken burgers

HEALTH BENEFITS
Chicken is a low-fat source of protein as long as the fatty skin is removed. It is also a good source of the amino acid tryptophan, which is vital for the production of the feel-good brain chemical serotonin.

Low in fat and high in protein, these chicken burgers are delicious cold and can be served either in a bun with relish and the usual accompaniments or solo with a dip such as Tzatziki (see page 34) or Tomato Salsa (see page 30). Instead of chicken, you could use turkey, lean beef or vegetarian mince.

1 small onion
2 tbsp chopped alfalfa sprouts
1 small carrot, finely grated
1 apple, cored, then grated,
    skin and all
450g/1lb chicken mince

1 small free-range egg,
    lightly beaten
plain flour, for dusting
salt
freshly ground black pepper
olive oil, for brushing

1 Put the onion, alfalfa sprouts, carrot, apple and mince in a mixing bowl. Stir or use your hands to break up the mince and mix everything together.

2 Add the egg and seasoning and mix again by hand.

3 Lightly cover a plate and your hands with flour. Divide the mince mixture into six and shape each portion into a round, flat burger. Place the burgers on a plate, cover with cling film and chill for 30 minutes.

4 Preheat the grill to medium and line a baking tray with foil. Lightly brush the foil with oil and place the burgers on top. Brush the top of the burgers with oil and grill for about 8 minutes on each side until golden.

MAKES 6

PREPARATION + COOKING
20 + 16 minutes + chilling

STORAGE
Make in advance and keep in the fridge for up to 3 days or freeze for up to 1 month (unless the chicken was frozen). Keep chilled until ready to eat (see page 17).

SERVE THIS WITH...
seeded burger bun
relish
tomato ketchup
lettuce and sliced tomato
Banana & Blueberry Muffin
  (see page 132)
fruit

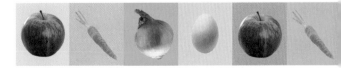

074

MAKES 6

PREPARATION + COOKING
10 + 12 minutes + chilling

STORAGE
Make in advance and keep in the fridge for up to 3 days or freeze for up to 1 month. Keep chilled until ready to eat (see page 17).

SERVE THIS WITH...
a bun (with favourite burger accompaniments) or on its own
Italian Flag Salad (see page 80)
Date & Pecan Brownie (see page 133)
fruit

HEALTH BENEFITS
Wholemeal bread is an unrefined carbohydrate food that contains plenty of fibre and will keep your child feeling fuller for longer than white bread would.

tuna patties

Canned tuna makes a convenient lunchbox staple, but instead of the usual sandwich filling here it is an ideal base for a pattie-cum-burger.

2 slices day-old
   wholemeal bread
200g/7oz canned lightmeat tuna
   in spring water, drained well
1 small onion, grated
1 tsp dried oregano
1 tbsp plain flour, plus extra
   for dusting
1 small free-range egg, beaten
salt
freshly ground black pepper
2 tbsp sunflower oil

1 Place the bread in a food processor or blender and process into breadcrumbs. Transfer to a mixing bowl with the tuna, onion, oregano, flour and egg. Season and chill for 1 hour to allow the mixture to firm up.

2 Lightly cover a plate and your hands in flour. Divide the tuna mixture into six and form into pattie shapes, then dust with more flour – the mixture is quite loose but will firm up when cooked.

3 Heat half of the oil in a frying pan and cook three of the patties for about 3 minutes on each side until golden, then drain on kitchen paper. Repeat with the remaining patties, adding more oil if necessary. Leave to cool before packing in an airtight container, placing a sheet of baking paper between each pattie.

courgette & parmesan fritters

These cheesy fritters taste delicious dipped into the Tomato Salsa on page 30. Lightly steamed chunks of broccoli, or peas or sweetcorn, can be used instead of the courgette, if preferred.

225g/8oz courgettes,
coarsely grated
3 tbsp finely grated
Parmesan cheese
1 free-range egg, beaten

2 tbsp white plain flour
2 tbsp sunflower oil
salt
freshly ground black pepper

1 Squeeze the courgettes in a tea-towel to remove any moisture. Mix the courgettes with the Parmesan, egg and flour, then season.

2 Heat half the oil in a frying pan. Add 2 tbsp courgette mixture for each fritter to make six in total. Cook in two batches for 2–3 minutes on each side until set and golden. Drain on kitchen paper and leave to cool.

MAKES 6

PREPARATION + COOKING
15 + 12 minutes

STORAGE
Make in advance and keep in the fridge for up to 3 days or freeze for up to 1 month.

SERVE THIS WITH...
Tortilla Dippers with Tomato Salsa (see page 30)
carrot and celery sticks
Cinnamon-spiced Apples (see page 120)

HEALTH BENEFITS
Summer squash such as courgettes are at their best during the warmer months; small ones have a better flavour than large ones.

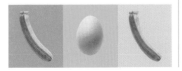

V O

spaghetti frittata

A great way to use up leftover spaghetti, this substantial "omelette" works well in a lunchbox, providing valuable amounts of both protein and carbohydrate.

SERVES 4–6

PREPARATION + COOKING
10 + 20 minutes

STORAGE
Make in advance and keep in the fridge for up to 3 days.

SERVE THIS WITH....
crusty bread
Mixed Bean Salad (see page 82)
muffin
fruit

HEALTH BENEFITS
Wholemeal or brown pasta is higher in fibre and B vitamins than the white varieties.

85g/3oz wholemeal or
    white spaghetti
olive oil, for stirring
5 free-range eggs, beaten

60g/2¼oz Parmesan
    cheese, grated
15g/½oz butter
salt
freshly ground black pepper

1 Cook the spaghetti in plenty of boiling water, following the packet instructions, until al dente. Drain and refresh under cold running water. Tip the pasta into a bowl, stir in a little oil to stop it sticking together, then leave to cool.
2 Season the beaten eggs and mix in the Parmesan. Preheat the grill to medium.
3 Melt the butter in a medium-sized frying pan with a heatproof handle. Place the spaghetti in the pan in an even layer, then pour the egg mixture over the pasta. Cook for about 5 minutes until the base is set and slightly golden.
4 Place the pan under the grill and cook the top of the frittata for about 3 minutes until set. Leave to cool, then cut into wedges.

tuna & onion tortilla

Substantial enough to withstand being carried about in a lunchbox, tortillas taste just as good cold as hot. A wedge of tortilla in a crusty roll with some chutney is a fine combination.

1 tbsp olive oil
1 large onion, sliced
200g/7oz canned lightmeat
  tuna, drained

450g/1lb cooked potatoes,
  peeled and diced
6 free-range eggs, beaten
salt
freshly ground black pepper

1 Heat the oil in a medium frying pan with a heatproof handle, then fry the onion for 8 minutes until softened and slightly golden. Stir in the tuna, retaining some chunks, then top with the potatoes, spreading the ingredients evenly.
2 Preheat the grill to medium. Season the eggs and pour them into the pan. Cook for 5 minutes over a medium heat until the base is golden and set.
3 Place the pan under the grill and cook the tortilla for about 3 minutes until set. Cool, then cut into wedges.

SERVES 4–6

PREPARATION + COOKING
10 + 17 minutes

STORAGE
Make in advance and keep in the fridge for up to 3 days. Keep chilled until ready to eat (see page 17).

SERVE THIS WITH…
Ham, Bean & Pineapple Salad
  (see page 84)
Carrot Cake (see page 134)
fruit

HEALTH BENEFITS
In natural medicine onions were praised as a "cure-all". Today they are believed to provide potent phytochemicals that may protect against both cancer and heart disease.

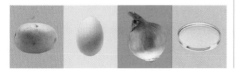

Ⓥ 🍽

vegetable samosas

Light and crisp low-fat filo pastry is used to make these lightly spiced Indian parcels.

MAKES 10

PREPARATION + COOKING
25 + 30 minutes

STORAGE
Make in advance and keep in the fridge for up to 3 days or freeze for up to 1 month.

SERVE THIS WITH...
Carrot, Raisin & Pinenut Salad (see page 77)
natural yogurt with honey
berries

HEALTH BENEFITS
Little nuggets of goodness, peas are a good source of protein, vitamins B and C, iron, potassium and phosphorus.

1 tbsp vegetable oil, plus extra
   for greasing
1 onion, finely chopped
1 carrot, diced
2 large cloves garlic,
   finely chopped
1 tbsp grated fresh ginger
2 tsp garam masala
¼ tsp chilli powder (optional)
250g/9oz cooked new
   potatoes, diced
3 tbsp frozen petits pois
salt
freshly ground black pepper
6 sheets filo pastry

1 Heat the oil in a frying pan and fry the onion for 3 minutes, then add the carrot and cook for another 4 minutes. Add the garlic, ginger and spices and cook for 1 more minute.
2 Stir in the potatoes, peas and 4 tbsp water, cover and simmer for 5 minutes to absorb the water. Season. Place in a bowl to cool. Preheat the oven to 190°C/375°F/Gas 5.
3 Lightly grease two baking trays. Take three sheets of filo pastry and place them on top of one another. Cut five 15cm/6in rounds and place on a baking sheet. Repeat.
4 Place a heaped tablespoon of filling in the centre of one round, wet the edge of the pastry and fold it over to make a half-moon shape, sealing the edges well. Brush with oil.
5 Repeat with the remaining rounds of filo and filling to make 10 samosas. Bake for 15 minutes until golden.

Ⓥ Ⓢ Ⓘ Ⓟ

spring rolls

Filled with crisp and crunchy vegetables, these spring rolls are baked to keep down fat levels.

55g/2oz rice vermicelli noodles
2 tsp sunflower oil, plus extra
   for brushing
1 tsp toasted sesame oil
2 carrots, cut into thin strips
1 red pepper, seeded and cut
   into thin strips
85g/3oz mangetout, sliced
   diagonally
2 cloves garlic, chopped

2 spring onions, finely
   sliced lengthways
2.5cm/1in piece fresh ginger,
   peeled and grated
2 tsp soy sauce
85g/3oz beansprouts
16 small spring roll wrappers,
   12cm/4½in square,
   defrosted if frozen
1 free-range egg white, beaten

1 Soak the noodles as instructed on the packet, drain and refresh under cold running water. Cut into short lengths.
2 Heat the oils in a wok and stir-fry the vegetables for 2 minutes. Add the soy sauce and cook for another minute. Add the beansprouts. Place in a bowl, stir and leave to cool.
3 Preheat the oven to 180°C/350°F/Gas 4. Put one wrapper at a time on a work surface (covering the rest with a damp tea towel). Place a heaped tablespoon of filling on one corner, fold the corner over it, fold in the two sides and roll the wrapper. Brush the edge with egg white and fold to seal.
4 Place the spring rolls on a lightly oiled baking tray. Brush each roll with oil and bake for 15 minutes until golden.

MAKES 16

PREPARATION + COOKING
25 + 20 minutes

STORAGE
Make in advance and keep in the fridge for up to 3 days or freeze for up to 1 month.

SERVE THIS WITH...
small pot of plum, soy or
  sweet chilli dipping sauce
Oriental Rice Salad (see page 91)
Apricot & Cashew Nut Bar
  (see page 128)
fruit

HEALTH BENEFITS
These spring rolls are an excellent way to encourage your child to eat a variety of vegetables. Try to provide a variety of coloured fresh veg, as each colour contains a range of healthy phytochemicals or plant nutrients.

*sushi cones

HEALTH BENEFITS
Sea vegetables such as nori are rich in minerals that benefit the nervous system, boost immunity and help the metabolism.

This may sound a bit complicated or indeed sophisticated for a child's lunchbox, but hand-rolled cones are surprisingly easy and don't need any specialist equipment. They're also fun to make and great for kids to get involved with. Instead of the hot-smoked trout or salmon, try slices of smoked trout, crabsticks, avocado, sweet pepper or cooked chicken.

100g/3½oz/½ cup sushi rice
1½ tbsp rice vinegar
½ tsp caster sugar
¼ tsp salt
3 sheets nori
2 tbsp mayonnaise
4 pea-sized amounts wasabi

80g/2¾oz hot-smoked trout or
    salmon, in large flakes
handful rocket leaves
6 thin sticks cucumber, seeded,
    5cm/2in long
tamari (wheat-free soy sauce)
    and pickled ginger, to serve
    (optional)

MAKES 6

PREPARATION + COOKING
25 + 15 minutes

STORAGE
Make the day before and keep in
the fridge overnight.

SERVE THIS WITH...
slices of sweet pepper and celery
Date & Pecan Brownie
 (see page 133)
fruit

1 Put the rice and 185ml/6fl oz/¾ cup water in a saucepan.
Bring to the boil, reduce to a simmer, cover and cook for
12–15 minutes until the water is absorbed. Leave for
5 minutes, covered.
2 Meanwhile, mix together the rice vinegar, sugar and salt.
Transfer the rice to a bowl to cool, then gently stir in the
rice vinegar mixture using a wooden spoon. Leave to cool.
3 Cut the nori sheets into six 10cm/4in squares. Mix the
mayonnaise and wasabi and smear over each square.
4 Place 2 tsp rice diagonally down the centre of each
square. On top lay a few flakes of trout, a few rocket
leaves and a stick of cucumber. Wet one edge of the nori
and roll into a cone shape; press the edge to seal.
5 Serve with tamari and pickled ginger, if liked.

Hot-smoked
fish has a more
delicate smoky
flavour than cold-
smoked fish, and
a firmer texture.

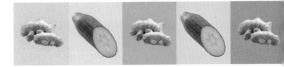

MAKES 8

PREPARATION + COOKING
10 + 20 minutes

STORAGE
Make in advance and keep in the fridge for up to 3 days or freeze for up to 1 month (unless the turkey was frozen). Keep chilled until ready to eat (see page 17).

SERVE THIS WITH…
Tortilla Dippers with Tomato Salsa (see page 30)
vegetable sticks
Winter Fruit Salad (see page 122)

HEALTH BENEFITS
An excellent low-fat source of protein, turkey also provides immune-boosting zinc as well as selenium.

festive turkey balls

These are very quick and simple to make and require a stuffing mix. The balls are an excellent filling for pitta bread or a tortilla wrap, or can be served on their own, dipped into the Tomato Salsa on page 30 or redcurrant sauce.

70g/2½oz good-quality organic stuffing mix
20g/¾oz unsalted butter

200g/7oz turkey breast, diced
olive oil, for brushing

1 Preheat the oven to 200°C/400°F/Gas 6. Make up the stuffing mix with 150ml/5fl oz/²/₃ cup just-boiled water and butter, following the packet instructions. Put the turkey in a food processor and process until very finely chopped. Add the stuffing mix and blend until combined.
2 Roll the mixture into eight balls slightly larger than a walnut and place in an oiled baking tin. Brush the balls with oil, then bake in the oven for about 20 minutes, turning occasionally, until golden and cooked through.

tandoori chicken drumsticks

Children love these lightly spiced chicken drumsticks, which can be eaten with their hands.

2 skinless chicken drumsticks
1 tbsp lemon juice
5 tbsp thick natural bio yogurt

2 tbsp tandoori spice blend
sunflower oil, for brushing

1 Pat the chicken dry with kitchen paper. Make three deep cuts in each drumstick and rub the lemon juice over them.
2 Put the yogurt and tandoori spices in a shallow dish and mix together. Add the chicken and completely cover with the marinade. Cover and chill for at least 1 hour.
3 Preheat the oven to 200°C/400°F/Gas 6. Brush a baking tray with oil and add the chicken. Cook in the oven for 15 minutes, then turn the chicken over and spoon over some more of the marinade. Cook for another 15 minutes until cooked through with no trace of pinkness inside.

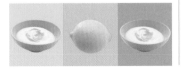

SERVES 2

PREPARATION + COOKING
15 + 30 minutes + marinating

STORAGE
Make the day before and keep in the fridge overnight. Keep chilled until ready to eat (see page 17).

SERVE THIS WITH...
Spicy Sweet Potatoes
(see page 95)
sliced cucumber
mango chutney
Banana & Blueberry Muffin
(see page 132)
fruit

HEALTH BENEFITS
Spices add plenty of flavour to food, but also have health benefits in that they help aid digestion and have valuable antibacterial properties.

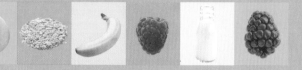

SWEET TREATS & BAKES

These desserts, cakes and breads have been created with health in mind – with a few concessions to the occasional indulgence. You'll find fresh and dried fruit in various guises, from fruit salads to muffins and cakes, and different takes on the cereal bar, including dates, apricots and cashews. Some of the sweet treats are sufficiently quick and simple to make on the day, while others need a bit more preparation but will keep for a few days. The Seeded Dough Balls, Cheese Scones and Oat Biscuits make a great alternative to bread while being just as versatile, and are perfect filled or topped with various sweet or savoury foods.

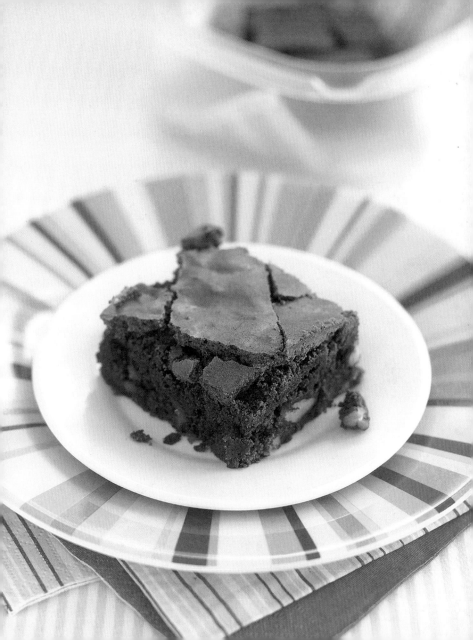

Ⓥ Ⓧ Ⓧ

cinnamon-spiced apples

SERVES 2–4

PREPARATION + COOKING
10 + 15 minutes

STORAGE
Make in advance and keep in the
fridge for up to 5 days or freeze
for up to 1 month.

SERVE THIS WITH...
Vegetable Samosas
  (see page 112)
Smashed Bean & Carrot Spread
  (see page 33)
vegetable sticks

HEALTH BENEFITS
In natural medicine, apples are
renowned for their cleansing
properties, and for their ability
to aid digestion and remove
impurities from the liver.

This lightly spiced apple compote can be
served on its own, stirred into vanilla custard
or puréed and combined with thick natural
yogurt. It freezes well, so can be prepared in
bulk and frozen in single portions for later use.

5 apples, cored, peeled and
  roughly chopped
1 tsp ground cinnamon

1 tsp fresh lemon juice
small knob of butter (optional)

1 Put the apples, cinnamon, lemon juice (this prevents the
apples turning brown), butter, if using, and 150ml/5fl oz/
²/₃ cup water in a saucepan. Bring to the boil, then simmer
over a medium-low heat for 12–15 minutes, until the
apples are tender.
2 Lightly mash the apples with a fork to break them down
slightly, then leave to cool.

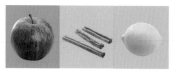

summer fruit salad

The beauty of a fruit salad is that it is infinitely flexible, allowing you to choose favourite fruits and the best of those in season. Try to use a variety of fruits of different shapes and colours, so that it will not only look good but also contain a range of nutrients.

8 strawberries, hulled and halved or quartered, if large
1 nectarine, stoned and cut into bite-sized chunks
1 kiwi fruit, peeled, quartered and cut into bite-sized chunks
1 apple, cored and cut into bite-sized chunks
8 seedless grapes, halved
4 tbsp orange juice

1 Divide the fruit between two lidded containers.
2 Pour 2 tbsp orange juice over each fruit salad and cover.

SERVES 2

PREPARATION
10 minutes

STORAGE
Make on the day itself for maximum nutrients or make the day before and keep overnight in the fridge.

SERVE THIS WITH...
Honey-sesame Sausages (see page 23)
Creamy Guacamole (see page 31)
pitta bread
vegetable sticks

HEALTH BENEFITS
Vitamin levels begin to deplete when fruit is cut, so it's best, if possible, to prepare fruit salad as close to serving as possible for maximum nutrient levels.

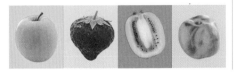

Ⓥ Ⓧ Ⓧ Ⓧ

winter fruit salad

With flavours reminiscent of Christmas, the cinnamon and cloves add a comforting warmth to this mineral-rich dried fruit salad. If your child finds chunks off-putting, the fruit salad can be puréed, with no ill effect on the taste, and mixed with natural yogurt.

SERVES 4

PREPARATION + COOKING
10 + 15 minutes

STORAGE
Make in advance and keep in the fridge for up to 1 week.

SERVE THIS WITH...
Festive Turkey Balls
 (see page 116)
wholemeal tortilla wrap
chutney
Cheesy Celery Sticks
 (see page 22)
cookie

HEALTH BENEFITS
Dried fruit has a rich concentration of beta-carotene, B vitamins, iron and potassium and is naturally sweet, so no extra sugar is needed.

200g/7oz mixed dried fruit such as apples, apricots, peaches and prunes, cut into bite-sized pieces
300ml/10fl oz/1¼ cup fresh orange juice

1 cinnamon stick
1 star anise
2 cloves

1 Put the dried fruit, orange juice, 6 tbsp water, cinnamon, star anise and cloves in a saucepan. Bring up to boiling point, then reduce the heat, cover and simmer for 10 minutes, until the fruit has softened.

2 Remove from the heat, leave to cool and divide between four small lidded pots.

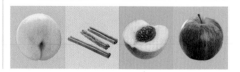

V ⊗ ⊗

mango fool

For the best-flavoured fool, make sure the mango is perfectly ripe and juicy. This creamy pudding is also delicious made with berries, plums or nectarines.

1 mango
100ml/3½fl oz/⅓ cup thick
  natural bio yogurt
150ml/5fl oz/⅔ cup low-fat
  fromage frais

1 tbsp clear honey, or to taste
1 tsp vanilla extract (optional)

1 Peel the mango using a vegetable peeler and slice the fruit off the large central stone. Put the mango in a blender with the rest of the ingredients and blend until smooth and creamy.
2 Transfer the mango fool to two lidded pots.

SERVES 2

PREPARATION
10 minutes

STORAGE
Make in advance and keep in the fridge for up to 3 days.

SERVE THIS WITH…
Chicken Tikka Naan (see page 66)
cucumber slices and
  cherry tomatoes
biscuit for dunking

HEALTH BENEFITS
An excellent source of vitamin C and beta-carotene, mango will benefit hair, skin and nails.

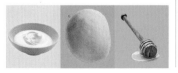

Ⓥ ⓧ ▷

*strawberry crunch pot

HEALTH BENEFITS
Energy-giving oats provide useful amounts of fibre and B vitamins. Research shows that foods high in carbohydrates boost the brain's levels of the feel-good chemical serotonin, levels of which tend to fall during the winter.

This is so simple to make and is much healthier than fruit yogurts from the shops – it is also an ideal breakfast or quick dessert. You could quadruple the oat and seed mixture, then store any surplus in an airtight jar for up to a week. If strawberries are out of season, sliced bananas are also good, or you could try frozen berries instead.

25g/1oz/¼ cup whole
  porridge oats
1 tbsp sunflower seeds
1 tbsp pumpkin seeds
1–2 tbsp clear honey or
  maple syrup

6 heaped tbsp thick natural
  bio yogurt
½ tsp vanilla extract
6 strawberries, hulled and
  thickly sliced

SERVES 1

PREPARATION + COOKING
10 + 5 minutes

STORAGE
Make the day before and keep
in the fridge overnight. The oat
and seed mixture will keep in an
airtight container for 1 week.

SERVE THIS WITH...
Creamy Tomato & Lentil Soup
  (see page 38)
bread
fruit

1 Put the oats in a dry frying pan and toast over a medium-low heat for 3 minutes, turning the oats occasionally with a spatula.

2 Next, add the sunflower and pumpkin seeds to the pan and toast for another 2 minutes, tossing the pan frequently until the oats and seeds are light golden.

3 Remove the pan from the heat and stir in the honey or maple syrup. This will sizzle at first, but keep stirring until the oats and seeds are coated. Leave to cool slightly to allow the mixture to crisp up.

4 Mix the yogurt with the vanilla extract.

5 Put a layer of the oat mixture in the bottom of a tall plastic pot. Top with half of the yogurt then half of the strawberries. Repeat with another layer of each. Cover.

**Honey is known
for its antiseptic
healing properties.
It's sweeter than
sugar so you
need less.**

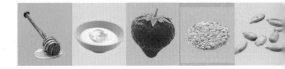

Ⓥ Ⓧ ▶

apple flapjacks

Full of energy-giving oats, fruit and seeds, these muesli-type bars are a perfect lunchbox treat.

MAKES 10

PREPARATION + COOKING
15 + 35 minutes

STORAGE
Make in advance and keep in an airtight container for up to 1 week.

SERVE THIS WITH....
Ham & Egg Pie (see page 103)
Carrot, Raisin & Pinenut Salad
(see page 77)
fruit

HEALTH BENEFITS
Pumpkin seeds are one of the few foods to contain both omega-3 and omega-6 essential fatty acids.

100g/3½oz unsalted butter,
    plus extra for greasing
100g/3½oz/scant ½ cup light
    soft brown sugar
4 tbsp golden syrup

250g/9oz/heaped 2 cups
    whole porridge oats
1 tbsp sesame seeds
1 tbsp pumpkin seeds
2 tbsp sunflower seeds
1 apple, cored and grated

1 Preheat the oven to 180°C/350°F/Gas 4. Grease the sides and line the base of a 20cm/8in square tin. Melt the butter in a saucepan with the sugar and syrup over a low heat, stirring occasionally; do not allow the mixture to boil.
2 Put the oats, seeds and apple in a mixing bowl and pour in the buttery syrup. Stir until everything is mixed together.
3 Spoon the oat mixture into the prepared tin and bake for 25–30 minutes until golden and lightly crisp. Cut into 10 bars while still warm and leave in the tin until cool.

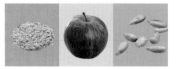

(V) (≥)

chewy date bars

Cereal bars can be on the dry side, but these have a layer of puréed dates for moistness.

125g/4½oz unsalted butter, plus extra for greasing
200g/7oz/1½ cups chopped ready-to-eat dried dates
125g/4½oz/1 cup wholemeal plain flour

1 tsp baking powder
115g/4oz/½ cup light soft brown sugar
125g/4½oz/generous cup whole porridge oats
4 tbsp sunflower seeds

1 Grease the sides and line the base of a 28 x 18cm/ 11 x 7in baking tin. Put the dates and 225ml/8fl oz/scant 1 cup water in a saucepan and bring to the boil. Reduce the heat and simmer, half-covered, for 20 minutes until the dates are very soft and the water has been absorbed. Purée the dates in a blender and leave to cool. Preheat the oven to 180°C/350°F/Gas 4.

2 Meanwhile, mix together the flour, baking powder, sugar, oats and seeds in a mixing bowl. Rub in the butter until the mixture is soft and crumbly. Spoon three-quarters into the greased tin and press down to make an even layer.

3 Spoon the date mixture over the oats in an even layer, sprinkle with the remaining oat mixture and press down lightly. Bake for 25 minutes until golden, then leave in the tin to cool. Cut into 16 squares and remove from the tin.

MAKES 16

PREPARATION + COOKING
20 + 45 minutes

STORAGE
Make in advance and keep in an airtight container for up to 1 week.

SERVE THIS WITH..
Spaghetti Frittata (see page 110) red pepper and celery sticks fruit

HEALTH BENEFITS
The brain needs a constant supply of glucose in order to function properly. Complex carbohydrates, found in the wholemeal flour and oats, are the primary source of the brain's energy.

Ⓥ Ⓧ 🍲 ⌀ ▷

apricot & cashew nut bars

These couldn't be simpler to make and are a wholesome blend of fruit, oats, nuts and seeds. Replace the nuts with more seeds, if necessary.

MAKES 8

PREPARATION + COOKING
10 + 3 minutes

STORAGE
Make in advance and keep in an airtight container for up to 1 week.

SERVE THIS WITH...
Sushi Cones (see page 114)
carrot sticks
fruit yogurt

HEALTH BENEFITS
Rich in B vitamins, vitamin E, iron, calcium, magnesium and potassium, cashew nuts provide numerous health benefits, but give them to your child in moderation because of their high fat content.

50g/2oz whole porridge oats
50g/2oz cashew nuts
150g/5½oz ready-to-eat dried unsulphured apricots, cut into small pieces

100g/3½oz raisins
4 tbsp fresh orange juice
2 tbsp sunflower seeds
2 tbsp pumpkin seeds

1 Put the oats and cashew nuts in a dry frying pan and toast them over a medium heat for 3 minutes, turning occasionally, until they start to turn golden. Leave to cool.

2 Put the apricots, raisins and orange juice in a food processor and process to a smooth paste. Scrape the fruit purée into a mixing bowl.

3 Put the oats, nuts and seeds in the food processor and process until finely chopped. Tip the mixture into the bowl with the fruit purée. Stir the fruit mixture until all the ingredients are mixed together.

4 Line an 18 x 25cm/7 x 10in tin with baking paper. Tip the mixture into the tin and smooth into an even layer about 1cm/½in thick. Chill for 1 hour, then cut into eight bars.

Ⓥ Ⓞ

drop scones with fruit sauce

Drop scones dipped into a smooth strawberry sauce are a great combination and fun to eat.

150g/5½oz/scant 1¼ cups
  self-raising flour
2 tsp caster sugar
200ml/7fl oz/generous
  ¾ cup milk
1 large free-range egg
vegetable oil, for frying

Fruit sauce:
300g/10½oz strawberries or
  mixture of berries
icing sugar, sifted, to taste

1 To make the fruit sauce, put the strawberries in a blender and process. Press the purée through a sieve into a bowl to remove any pips, and sweeten with icing sugar to taste.
2 To make the drop scones, sift the flour into a mixing bowl, then mix with the sugar. Make a well in the centre. Pour the milk into a jug, whisk in the egg, then add to the flour and sugar. Beat to make a smooth batter.
3 Heat a little oil in a non-stick frying pan and add three small ladlefuls of batter, one for each drop scone. Cook for about 3 minutes until light golden, then turn and cook for another 2 minutes. Remove and cook the remaining scones.
4 Put the fruit sauce into individual lidded pots.

MAKES 10 (2 PER PERSON)

PREPARATION + COOKING
10 + 20 minutes

STORAGE
Make in advance and keep in the fridge for up to 3 days or freeze for up to 1 month.

SERVE THIS WITH...
Sweetcorn Chowder
  (see page 40)
crusty bread
fruit

HEALTH BENEFITS
Strawberries help to boost the immune system thanks to their collection of potent antioxidants. As the fruit sauce is uncooked, the high levels of vitamin C will remain intact.

HEALTH BENEFITS
Berries are an excellent source of vitamin C, folate and the antioxidants ellagic acid and quercetin. They are also thought to help prevent cold sores, asthma and hay fever.

summer puddings

Packed with juicy summer berries, these little summer puddings don't just look good: they're full of vitamins too. You could use fresh berries, but frozen bags of mixed fruit mean that you can make these fruity puddings at any time of year.

vegetable oil, for greasing
10–12 thin small slices
    wholemeal bread,
    crusts removed

2 x 500g/1lb 2oz/10-cup bags
    frozen summer berries
6 tbsp caster sugar

SERVES 4

PREPARATION + COOKING
15 + 5 minutes

STORAGE
Make in advance and keep in the
fridge for up to 3 days or freeze
for up to 1 month.

SERVE THIS WITH...
Tuna Quesadilla (see page 65)
cucumber and cherry tomatoes

1 Lightly oil four 150ml/5fl oz dariole moulds or small
lidded pots. Cut four circles of bread to fit the base of each
mould. Cut each of the remaining bread slices into four
triangles. Put a bread round into each mould, then arrange
the triangular pieces of bread around the sides, packing
them tightly together to avoid any gaps. Allow the bread
to overlap the top slightly. Set aside four triangles.
2 Meanwhile, put the fruit in a saucepan with the sugar
and 120ml/4fl oz/½ cup water and simmer gently for 4–5
minutes until the berries are defrosted and very juicy.
3 Spoon a little of the berry juice into each mould, then
divide the fruit between the moulds, leaving 4 tbsp juice
to spoon over the puddings.
4 Fold the bread over the fruit filling, then top with the
remaining triangles. Spoon over the juice, then cover each
pudding with a plate and a weight and refrigerate overnight.

Among their many
health benefits,
berries are a good
source of lutein,
which is important
for healthy vision.

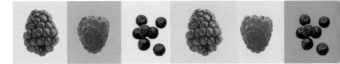

MAKES 10

PREPARATION + COOKING
15 + 20 minutes

STORAGE
Make the day before and keep in an airtight container. Muffins are best eaten as fresh as possible.

SERVE THIS WITH…
Chicken Strips with Satay Dip (see page 26)
pitta bread
carrot sticks and cherry tomatoes
fruit

HEALTH BENEFITS
A superfood, blueberries are rich in powerful antioxidants called anthocyanins, which mop up potentially harmful free radicals in the body.

Ⓥ Ⓞ

banana & blueberry muffins

These muffins will give pre-lunch depleted blood-sugar levels a welcome boost.

225g/8oz/1¾ cups white
  plain flour
pinch of salt
1 tsp baking powder
150g/5oz/⅔ cup caster sugar
100ml/3½fl oz/⅓ cup milk

2 free-range eggs
150g/5oz unsalted butter,
  melted
2 bananas, mashed
150g/5½oz/1 cup blueberries

1 Preheat the oven to 200°C/400°F/Gas 6. Place 10 large paper cases in a deep muffin tin.
2 Sift the flour, salt and baking powder into a mixing bowl, stir in the sugar and mix together. Make a well in the centre.
3 Put the milk, eggs and butter in a jug and whisk until combined. Add to the bowl with the bananas, stir just to combine, then fold in the blueberries. Spoon into the tin.
4 Bake for 20 minutes until risen. Cool on a wire rack.

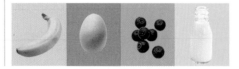

Ⓥ Ⓞ ⦿

date & pecan brownies

These fruit-and-nut chocolate brownies make a perfect treat. Leave the pecans out if necessary.

100g/3½oz/1 cup pecans,
 broken in half
150g/5½oz dark chocolate,
 broken into chunks
150g/5½oz unsalted butter,
 cut into pieces
280g/10oz/1¼ cups
 caster sugar

3 free-range eggs,
 lightly beaten
125g/4½oz/1 cup white
 plain flour
1½ tsp baking powder
100g/3½oz dried ready-to-eat
 dates, cut into small pieces

1 Preheat the oven to 180°C/350°F/Gas 4. Line and grease a 20cm/8in square cake tin. Put the pecans on a baking tray and roast for about 5 minutes until they are slightly golden and smell toasted.

2 Meanwhile, melt the chocolate and butter in a bowl over a pan of slightly simmering water, stirring very occasionally. Remove from the heat and leave to cool slightly.

3 Whisk together the sugar and eggs in a bowl until pale, and stir into the chocolate mixture. Sift in the flour and baking powder, then add the pecans and dates. Mix with a wooden spoon, then pour the mixture into the cake tin.

4 Cook for 40–45 minutes until the top forms a light crust, but the centre is still slightly gooey. Leave to cool in the tin, then turn out and cut into 12 squares.

MAKES 12

PREPARATION + COOKING
15 + 50 minutes

STORAGE
Make in advance and keep in an airtight container for up to 1 week.

SERVE THIS WITH...
Cheese, Apple & Chutney Bap
 (see page 52)
carrot and pepper sticks
fruit

HEALTH BENEFITS
Dates are a rich source of fibre, are high in potassium and contain some iron, while pecans contain protein, iron, calcium and fibre.

095

Ⓥ Ⓞ ⓑ

carrot cake

This is one of the easiest cakes in the world to make, but it's still incredibly light and moist.

MAKES 15 SQUARES

PREPARATION + COOKING
20 + 50 minutes

STORAGE
Make in advance and keep in an airtight container for up to 1 week.

SERVE THIS WITH...
Sweetcorn Chowder
(see page 40)
wholemeal pitta bread
fruit

HEALTH BENEFITS
Recent research has found that, along with bountiful amounts of beneficial nutrients, carrots may help to protect against food poisoning.

butter, for greasing
125g/4½oz/1 cup wholemeal
   self-raising flour
125g/4½oz/1 cup white self-
   raising flour
2 tsp ground mixed spice
250g/9oz/heaped 1 cup light
   soft brown sugar
250g/9oz carrots, grated

4 free-range eggs, lightly beaten
200ml/7fl oz/generous ¾ cup
   sunflower oil

Icing:
125g/4½oz/½ cup low-fat
   cream cheese
5 tbsp icing sugar
1 tsp vanilla extract

1 Preheat the oven to 180°C/350°F/Gas 4. Grease the sides and line the base of a 20cm/8in square cake tin.
2 Sift the flours into a mixing bowl, adding the bran left in the sieve. Stir in the spice, sugar and carrots and thoroughly combine.
3 Add the eggs and oil, then stir until all the ingredients are combined. Pour into the tin and smooth the top. Bake for 50 minutes until risen and golden. Leave in the tin for 10 minutes, then turn out on to a rack and leave to cool.
4 Beat the cream cheese and icing sugar in a mixing bowl until smooth and creamy. Stir in the vanilla extract. Chill for 10 minutes, then spread over the cake and smooth with a palette knife. Cut into 15 squares.

(V) (O)

custard tartlets

These mini custard tarts make a great treat in a lunchbox. What's more, the pastry is filo, which is lower in fat than shortcrust or puff and needs no preparation.

3 sheets filo pastry, defrosted
  if frozen
20g/¾oz butter, melted
2 large free-range eggs

3 tbsp caster sugar
300ml/10fl oz/1¼ cups milk
1 tsp vanilla extract
freshly grated nutmeg

1 Preheat the oven to 190°C/375°F/Gas 5. Place the sheets of filo on top of one another and cut into eight 11cm/4½in squares.

2 Lightly brush eight holes of a deep muffin tin with melted butter, then place a three-layered square of filo pastry in each one. Press the filo into each hole, leaving the top to overhang the tin. Brush the top of the filo with the rest of the melted butter.

3 Whisk together the eggs and sugar in a bowl. Heat the milk, then pour it into the egg mixture with the vanilla and whisk again. Strain the mixture into a jug, then pour into the pastry cases. Grate a little nutmeg over the top.

4 Bake the tartlets for about 20 minutes until the pastry is golden and the filling set. Transfer to a wire rack to cool.

MAKES 8

PREPARATION + COOKING
10 + 20 minutes

STORAGE
Make in advance and keep in the fridge for up to 3 days.

SERVE THIS WITH…
Pesto Pasta Salad (see page 86)
fruit

HEALTH BENEFITS
Eggs are packed with nutrients, including protein, vitamins A, D, E and the B group, as well as the minerals iron, phosphorus and zinc.

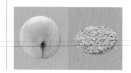

apricot cookies

These moreish American-style cookies contain nutritious oats and apricots.

MAKES 10

PREPARATION + COOKING
15 + 20 minutes

STORAGE
Make in advance and keep in an airtight container for up to 1 week.

SERVE THIS WITH…
Tandoori Chicken Drumstick (see page 117)
naan bread
green salad
fruit

HEALTH BENEFITS
Try to use unsulphured dried apricots. These are darker in colour and don't contain the preservative sulphur, which asthma sufferers should avoid.

70g/2½oz light soft brown sugar
125g/4½oz unsalted butter, softened and cubed
70g/2½oz/½ cup white self-raising flour
30g/1oz/¼ cup wholemeal self-raising flour
100g/3½oz/1 cup porridge oats
5 ready-to-eat dried apricots, cut into small pieces

1 Preheat the oven to 180°C/350°F/Gas 4. Line two baking trays with baking paper.
2 Cream the sugar and butter together in a mixing bowl until light and fluffy. Fold in both types of flour, the oats and apricots and beat until creamy.
3 Divide the mixture into 10 pieces and roll each one into a ball. Arrange on the prepared baking trays, well spaced out to allow for the cookies to spread. Flatten the top of each ball slightly and bake for 15–20 minutes until just golden but still slightly soft in the centre.
4 Transfer the cookies to a wire rack to cool.

Ⓥ

oat biscuits

These biscuits are very popular served on their own, spread with jam or cream cheese, or with a chunk of cheese or slice of ham.

vegetable oil, for greasing
50g/1¾oz/½ cup
    medium oatmeal
85g/3oz/²/₃ cup wholemeal plain
    flour, plus extra for dusting

1 tsp baking powder
pinch of salt
50g/1¾oz butter, diced
1 tbsp caster sugar
2 tbsp milk

1 Preheat the oven to 200°C/400°F/Gas 6. Lightly grease a baking tray.

2 Sift the oatmeal, flour and baking powder into a mixing bowl, adding any bran left in the sieve. Add the salt and stir until combined.

3 Rub the butter and sugar into the flour mixture, using fingertips, until it resembles breadcrumbs. Pour in the milk and mix with a fork and then your hands to make a dough.

4 Turn the dough on to a lightly floured work surface and knead briefly until smooth. Using a floured rolling pin, roll out the dough into a rectangle about 5mm/¼in thick. Trim the edges and cut into 12 squares, re-rolling as necessary.

5 Place the oat biscuits on the baking tray and prick the top of the biscuits with a fork. Bake for 10 minutes until light golden. Transfer to a wire rack to cool.

MAKES 12

PREPARATION + COOKING
15 + 10 minutes

STORAGE
Make in advance and keep in an airtight container for up to 1 week.

SERVE THIS WITH...
chunk of cheese or slice of ham
Creamy Tomato & Lentil Soup
 (see page 38)
fruit yogurt
fruit

HEALTH BENEFITS
Oats are a low-GI complex carbohydrate, meaning that they are absorbed slowly into the bloodstream and have a stabilizing effect on blood-sugar levels, thus ensuring sustained amounts of energy.

V O

cheese scones

Savoury scones make a tasty alternative to sandwiches in a lunchbox. These cheesy ones are good on their own or with soup or a salad. Alternatively, fill with crispy bacon, ham, cream cheese and chives or a filling of your choice.

MAKES 10

PREPARATION
10 + 12 minutes

STORAGE
Make in advance and keep in an airtight container for up to 3 days or freeze for up to 1 month.

SERVE THIS WITH…
Creamy Tomato & Lentil Soup (see page 38)
Apricot & Cashew Nut Bar (see page 128)
fruit

HEALTH BENEFITS
Extra-virgin olive oil is used instead of butter to make these scones, providing beneficial monounsaturated fat rather than saturated fat. Monounsaturated fat does not lower blood cholesterol but is good at maintaining levels of "good" cholesterol in the body.

150g/5½oz/1¼ cups white self-raising flour
70g/2½oz/½ cup wholemeal self-raising flour
½ tsp baking powder
90g/3½oz mature Cheddar cheese, grated
2 tbsp extra-virgin olive oil
6–7 tbsp milk, plus extra for brushing
1 large free-range egg, beaten

1 Preheat the oven to 220°C/425°F/Gas 7. Lightly dust a baking tray with flour. Sift both types of flour and baking powder into a mixing bowl, adding any bran left in the sieve. Stir in the Cheddar and make a well in the centre.
2 Pour in the oil, milk and egg and mix with a palette knife to form a soft dough. Add a little extra milk if the dough seems dry. Transfer the dough to a lightly floured work surface and knead briefly until smooth.
3 Roll out the dough into a rectangle about 2.5cm/1in thick, then cut into 10. Arrange the scones on the baking tray and brush the tops with a little milk. Bake for 10–12 minutes until risen and golden.

Ⓥ ⊖ ⊘

seeded dough balls

Dunk these into soup, hummus, guacamole or a bean dip or serve with a salad.

350ml/12fl oz/1½ cups
   tepid water
2 tsp dried yeast
350g/12oz/3 cups strong white
   bread flour

150g/5½oz/1¼ cups strong
   wholemeal bread flour
1½ tsp salt
5 tbsp toasted sunflower seeds
olive oil, for brushing

1 Pour 6 tbsp of water into a small bowl. Sprinkle in the yeast, stir until dissolved and set aside for 5 minutes. Sift the flours and salt into a large bowl. Stir in the seeds.
2 Make a well in the centre of the flour and pour in the yeast mixture and 250ml/9fl oz/1 cup water. Gradually stir in the flour from the sides of the well. Stir in 3–4 tbsp water, if necessary, to make a soft dough.
3 Turn the dough out on to a lightly floured work surface. Knead for 10 minutes until smooth and elastic. Put in a new bowl and cover with a tea towel. Leave for 1½–2 hours.
4 Preheat the oven to 220°C/425°F/Gas 7. Press the dough with your knuckles, then divide into 20 pieces. Flatten each piece slightly, fold it over, then roll into a ball in your palm. Place on a floured baking sheet and leave for 10 minutes.
5 Brush with olive oil and bake for 15–20 minutes until risen and golden. Cool on a wire rack.

MAKES 20

PREPARATION + COOKING
25 + 20 minutes + rising

STORAGE
Make in advance and keep in an airtight container for up to 5 days or freeze for up to 1 month.

SERVE THIS WITH...
Italian Flag Salad (see page 80)
carrot sticks
Summer Fruit Salad
  (see page 121)

HEALTH BENEFITS
Omega-6 essential fatty acids, calcium, zinc, magnesium and vitamin E are found in beneficial amounts in sunflower seeds.

menu plans

wheat- & gluten-free 5-day menu

A wheat- and gluten-free diet was once thought to be restrictive and nutrient-deficient, but we now have a greater understanding of special dietary needs, and food manufacturers are offering far more choice than before. Some sauces and condiments are unsuitable, so check labels.

Day 1
Tuna & Onion Tortilla (see page 111)
wheat-/gluten-free wholemeal bread
red pepper and cucumber sticks
Summer Fruit Salad (see page 121)

Day 2
Rice Paper Rolls (see page 73)
Super Salad (see page 81)
Mango Fool (see page 123)
fruit

Day 3
Smoked Mackerel, Apple & Potato Salad
(see page 96)
wheat-/gluten-free crackers

chunk of cheese
natural yogurt and honey
fruit

Day 4
Melon & Halloumi Salad (see page 78)
wheat-/gluten-free flatbread
vegetable sticks, such as carrot, pepper,
cucumber or celery
Winter Fruit Salad (see page 122)

Day 5
Spicy Carrot & Lentil Soup (see page 41)
Pear & Ham Bundles (see page 24)
wheat-/gluten-free wholemeal roll
fruit

vegetarian 5-day menu

This menu follows the basic principles of a vegetarian diet: to avoid meat, poultry and fish and any food that contains ingredients derived from an animal, such as gelatine in jelly or animal rennet in some cheeses.

Day 1
Creamy Tomato & Lentil Soup (see page 38)
Seeded Dough Balls (see page 139) or bread
chunk of vegetarian cheese
Banana & Blueberry Muffin (see page 132)
grapes

Day 2
Vegetable Samosa (see page 112)
Carrot, Raisin & Pinenut Salad (see page 77)
Cinnamon-spiced Apples (see page 120)
milk

Day 3
Spaghetti Frittata (see page 110)
Tortilla Dippers with Tomato Salsa
  (see page 30)

green salad
Apricot Cookies (see page 136)
fruit

Day 4
Bbq Tofu Baguette (see page 54)
Creamy Guacamole (see page 31)
vegetable sticks
natural yogurt with honey
fruit

Day 5
Falafel & Hummus Lavash (see page 68)
Tabbouleh (see page 90)
carrot sticks
fruit
chocolate milk

vegan 5-day menu

This menu follows the basic principles of a vegan diet: to avoid any animal-derived food, such as meat, poultry and seafood, as well as ingredients that are a by-product of animals, including dairy produce and honey. This does not mean that a vegan diet is restrictive, but you need to ensure that your child is getting a healthy mix of vital nutrients.

Day 1
Soy-coated Nuts & Seeds (see page 20)
Miso & Tofu Broth (see page 43), using
    rice noodles
Apricot & Cashew Nut Bar (see page 128)
fruit

Day 2
Bbq Tofu Baguette (see page 54), using
    maple syrup/sweet chilli sauce instead
    of honey
cherry tomatoes
Winter Fruit Salad (see page 122)

Day 3
Roasted Red Pepper Hummus
    (see page 28)
breadsticks
selection of vegetable sticks

Savoury Spicy Popcorn (see page 21)
soya yogurt
fruit

Day 4
Spicy Bulghur Salad with Nectarines
    (see page 92)
Smashed Bean & Carrot Spread
    (see page 33)
pitta bread
fruit

Day 5
Vegetable Samosa (see page 112)
Spicy Sweet Potatoes (see page 95),
    using soya yogurt
Apple Flapjack (see page 126), using
    vegetable margarine instead of butter
fruit

nut-free 5-day menu

One in six people in the UK suffer from some form of allergy, and an allergy to nuts is becoming increasingly common. As the symptoms of this allergy are usually life-threatening, it's vital that nut-allergy sufferers avoid any contact with nuts and by-products, which is why many schools now have a ban on nuts and related foods. Always check food labels.

Day 1

Smashed Bean & Carrot Spread
(see page 33)
chunk of cheese
Oat Biscuit (see page 137)
cherry tomatoes
Summer Fuit Salad (see page 121)

Day 2

Chicken Noodle Soup (see page 46)
wholemeal bread
Custard Tartlet (see page 135)
fruit

Day 3

Sardines & Tomato on Brown (see page 57)
Apple Coleslaw (see page 76)
natural yogurt with honey
fruit

Day 4

Sausage & Barley Salad (see page 94)
carrot sticks
hard-boiled egg
fruit

Day 5

Calzone (see page 101)
green salad
Banana & Blueberry Muffin (see page 132)
fruit

INDEX